LIVING WITH

DIABETES

as a SENIOR

Empowering Wellness and Independence: Navigating Diabetes with Wisdom and Grace in the Golden Years

Catherine CLARKSON

Contents

Introduction

Embracing Life with Diabetes as a Senior

Welcome to a journey of empowerment and resilience – a guide crafted specifically for seniors navigating the complex terrain of diabetes. In the golden years of life, the challenges posed by diabetes can seem formidable. Still, this book aims to be your steadfast companion, providing knowledge, support, and practical strategies to not just manage, but truly embrace life with diabetes.

As a senior facing the realities of diabetes, you may find yourself at a crossroads of uncertainty. But fear not; this book is here to illuminate the path ahead. It recognizes the unique nuances of managing diabetes in your later years, addressing the physical, emotional, and practical aspects with compassion and understanding.

The term 'embracing' is intentionally chosen to signify a proactive and positive approach to living with diabetes. Rather than merely coping or enduring, we invite you to embrace the opportunities for growth, self-care, and joy that can coexist with diabetes. This journey is not just about managing blood sugar levels; it's about embracing a fulfilling and vibrant life despite the challenges.

Through these pages, we will delve into the intricacies of understanding diabetes in seniors, exploring lifestyle modifications, decoding medications and insulin management, and unraveling the mysteries of monitoring blood sugar levels. Moreover, we will shine a light on preventing and managing complications, fostering a strong support system, and navigating the emotional landscape often accompanying this journey.

Each chapter is a stepping stone, guiding you towards a holistic approach to diabetes care tailored to the senior experience. Drawing from a wealth of knowledge, practical advice, and the shared experiences of others who have walked this path, we aim to empower you to make informed decisions about your health, foster a sense of control, and ultimately, enhance your quality of life.

So, let's embark on this journey together – a journey of embracing life with diabetes as a senior. May this book be a source of inspiration, resilience, and a reminder that with the right tools and mindset, life can be not just managed, but truly celebrated.

Chapter 1:

Understanding Diabetes in Seniors

Diabetes, a complex and pervasive health condition, touches the lives of millions worldwide. As we age into our senior years, the impact of diabetes becomes increasingly profound, demanding a deeper understanding of its intricacies and nuances. This chapter serves as a comprehensive exploration of diabetes in seniors, covering key aspects such as the general overview of the condition, its prevalence in the senior population, and the various types of diabetes that can manifest in this demographic.

1.1 Overview of Diabetes

Diabetes, often described as a metabolic disorder, is characterized by elevated blood glucose levels resulting from the body's inability to produce or effectively use insulin. This hormone, produced by the pancreas, plays a crucial role in regulating blood sugar levels. Without proper insulin function, glucose builds up in the bloodstream, leading to a myriad of health complications.

In seniors, the impact of diabetes is magnified, requiring a nuanced understanding of the condition's implications on overall health and well-being. The most common types of diabetes include Type 1, Type 2, and gestational diabetes, each with distinct characteristics and underlying causes.

Type 1 diabetes, typically diagnosed in childhood or adolescence, occurs when the immune system mistakenly attacks and destroys the insulin-producing cells in the pancreas. Seniors can also develop Type 1 diabetes, although it is less common in this age group.

Type 2 diabetes, on the other hand, is the more prevalent form, especially among seniors. It results from insulin resistance, where the body's cells don't respond effectively to insulin, leading to an insulin production overload. Factors such as genetics, sedentary lifestyle, and obesity play significant roles in the development of Type 2 diabetes.

Gestational diabetes manifests during pregnancy and increases the risk of Type 2 diabetes later in life. While not exclusive to seniors, understanding its implications is vital for comprehensive diabetes awareness.

The impact of diabetes extends beyond the immediate concern of blood sugar management. It affects various organs and systems, including the heart, kidneys, eyes, and nervous system. Seniors, often managing multiple health issues concurrently, face unique challenges in balancing diabetes care with other aspects of their well-being.

A holistic approach to diabetes in seniors encompasses not only blood glucose monitoring and medication management but also lifestyle adjustments, nutritional considerations, and a keen awareness of potential complications. The journey of understanding diabetes starts with grasping its fundamental nature, its impact on seniors, and the multi-faceted strategies needed for effective management.

1.2 Prevalence in the Senior Population

As the global population ages, the prevalence of diabetes among seniors has reached alarming levels, transforming it into a major public health concern. Understanding the scope of this issue is crucial for healthcare professionals, caregivers, and seniors themselves. The rise in diabetes prevalence among seniors is influenced by a combination of demographic shifts, lifestyle factors, and the physiological changes that accompany aging.

Demographically, the aging population is growing at an unprecedented rate. Improved healthcare and advances in medical science have contributed to increased life expectancy, leading to a larger proportion of seniors in the overall population. With this demographic shift comes an increased susceptibility to chronic health conditions, including diabetes.

Lifestyle factors play a pivotal role in the prevalence of diabetes among seniors. Sedentary lifestyles, unhealthy dietary habits, and obesity are significant contributors. Seniors may face challenges in maintaining an active lifestyle due to physical limitations, and dietary choices can be influenced by factors such as accessibility, affordability, and changes in taste perception.

Physiological changes associated with aging also contribute to the increased prevalence of diabetes. Insulin resistance tends to rise with age, making seniors more susceptible to Type 2 diabetes. Additionally, hormonal changes, especially in postmenopausal women, can impact blood sugar regulation.

It is essential to recognize the diversity within the senior population concerning diabetes prevalence. Factors such as ethnicity, socioeconomic status, and geographic location can influence the likelihood of developing diabetes. Tailoring awareness campaigns and healthcare interventions to address these diverse needs is crucial for effective diabetes management among seniors.

The consequences of unmanaged diabetes in seniors are severe and far-reaching. Increased risk of cardiovascular diseases, kidney complications, vision problems, and neuropathy are just a few of the potential outcomes. Understanding the prevalence of diabetes in the senior population is the first step in developing targeted strategies for prevention, early detection, and comprehensive management.

1.3 Types of Diabetes in Seniors

Seniors, like individuals of any age group, can experience different types of diabetes, each presenting its own set of challenges and considerations. Understanding the nuances of these diabetes types is essential for tailored and effective management in the senior population.

Type 1 Diabetes in Seniors: While commonly associated with children and young adults, Type 1 diabetes can also affect seniors. This form of diabetes results from the immune system mistakenly attacking the insulin-producing cells in the pancreas. Seniors diagnosed with Type 1 diabetes often face unique challenges, as this condition requires lifelong insulin therapy and vigilant management.

Type 2 Diabetes in Seniors: The most prevalent form of diabetes among seniors is Type 2 diabetes. It typically develops due to insulin resistance, where the body's cells do not respond effectively to insulin. Age-related factors, such as decreased physical activity, changes in metabolism, and increased prevalence of obesity, contribute to the higher incidence of

Type 2 diabetes in seniors. Management involves lifestyle modifications, oral medications, and, in some cases, insulin therapy.

Gestational Diabetes and its Relevance in Seniors: Gestational diabetes, a condition that occurs during pregnancy, can have implications for seniors. Women who have gestational diabetes may have an increased risk of developing Type 2 diabetes later in life. Understanding this connection is crucial for seniors, especially women, as it underscores the importance of ongoing monitoring and preventive measures.

Other Types of Diabetes in Seniors: Beyond Type 1 and Type 2, seniors may also experience other forms of diabetes, including monogenic diabetes and secondary diabetes due to certain medications or underlying health conditions. Each type requires a tailored approach to management, considering the specific factors influencing blood sugar regulation.

It is paramount for seniors and their healthcare providers to recognize the unique characteristics of each diabetes type. Tailoring management plans to address individual needs, considering factors such as overall health, lifestyle, and potential complications, is crucial for optimal outcomes.

Understanding the types of diabetes that can affect seniors is the foundation for effective management. This knowledge empowers seniors to actively participate in their care, make informed decisions, and work collaboratively with healthcare professionals to enhance their overall well-being.

Chapter 2:

Managing Diabetes Through Lifestyle Changes

Diabetes management among seniors goes beyond medications and insulin therapy; it involves embracing lifestyle changes that can significantly impact overall well-being. In this chapter, we delve into the crucial role of lifestyle adjustments, with a specific focus on the importance of a healthy diet. Understanding how dietary choices influence blood sugar levels is fundamental, and we explore the intricacies of choosing the right foods, effective meal planning, and mastering portion control to foster sustainable and positive changes in the senior diabetic journey.

2.1 Importance of a Healthy Diet

The adage "you are what you eat" holds profound significance, especially for seniors managing diabetes. A healthy diet is not just a component of diabetes management; it is a cornerstone, influencing blood sugar levels, energy levels, and overall health. In the context of senior citizens, the importance of a healthy diet takes on added significance, considering the unique nutritional needs and challenges that come with aging.

For seniors with diabetes, a healthy diet serves as a powerful tool to regulate blood sugar levels, prevent complications, and contribute to an enhanced quality of life. The components of a diabetes-friendly diet extend beyond simply controlling carbohydrates; it involves a balanced and nutrient-dense approach that addresses the specific needs of seniors.

Understanding the key elements of a healthy diet for seniors with diabetes involves exploring the role of macronutrients (carbohydrates, proteins, and fats), micronutrients (vitamins and minerals), and dietary fiber. Each plays a crucial role in maintaining optimal health and supporting diabetes management.

Balancing Carbohydrates: Carbohydrates have a direct impact on blood sugar levels, making their management central to diabetes care. However, it is not about eliminating carbohydrates but making wise choices. Seniors are encouraged to focus on complex carbohydrates, such as whole grains, vegetables, and legumes, which release glucose into the bloodstream more slowly, preventing sharp spikes.

Proteins for Sustained Energy: Proteins play a crucial role in providing sustained energy and supporting muscle health, which is particularly important for seniors. Sources of lean protein, such as poultry, fish, beans, and tofu, should be incorporated into meals to promote overall well-being.

Healthy Fats for Heart Health: Including healthy fats in the diet is essential for seniors, especially given the increased risk of cardiovascular complications. Opting for sources of unsaturated fats, such as avocados, nuts, and olive oil, supports heart health while providing a satisfying and flavorful component to meals.

Micronutrients and Antioxidants: Seniors need a diverse range of vitamins and minerals to support various bodily functions. A diet rich in colorful fruits and vegetables ensures an ample supply of antioxidants, which protect cells from damage and contribute to overall health.

Dietary Fiber for Digestive Health: Adequate dietary fiber is crucial for seniors, as it aids in digestion, helps manage blood sugar levels, and supports heart health. Whole grains, fruits, vegetables, and legumes are excellent sources of fiber that seniors can incorporate into their meals.

Hydration: Proper hydration is often overlooked but is a critical aspect of a healthy diet. Seniors with diabetes should be mindful of their fluid intake, choosing water as the primary beverage and avoiding sugary drinks.

Tailoring a healthy diet to the specific needs of seniors with diabetes involves individualized considerations. Factors such as existing health conditions, medications, and personal preferences should be taken into account when crafting a nutrition plan. Consulting with a healthcare professional or a registered dietitian is recommended to develop a personalized and sustainable dietary approach.

2.1.1 Choosing the Right Foods

The concept of choosing the right foods transcends a mere list of dos and don'ts; it involves cultivating a mindful and informed approach to nutrition. Seniors with diabetes are empowered when equipped with knowledge about the impact of different foods on their blood sugar levels. Making informed choices is not about deprivation but rather about making conscious decisions that contribute to overall well-being.

Low-Glycemic Foods: Understanding the glycemic index (GI) is a valuable tool for seniors with diabetes. Foods with a low GI release glucose slowly into the bloodstream, preventing rapid spikes in blood sugar levels. Opting for whole grains, non-starchy vegetables, and legumes can be beneficial for seniors seeking stable and sustained energy.

Lean Proteins: Including lean protein sources in the diet is essential for seniors, supporting muscle health and providing a feeling of satiety. Fish, poultry, tofu, legumes, and low-fat dairy products are excellent choices. These foods contribute to overall nutritional balance without significantly affecting blood sugar levels.

Healthy Fats: Seniors should focus on incorporating sources of healthy fats into their diet, promoting heart health, and adding flavor to meals. Avocados, nuts, seeds, and olive oil are examples of unsaturated fats that can be included in moderation.

Colorful Fruits and Vegetables: The vibrant hues of fruits and vegetables indicate a rich array of nutrients and antioxidants. Seniors are encouraged to consume a variety of colorful produce to ensure they receive a diverse range of vitamins, minerals, and protective compounds.

Whole Grains: Choosing whole grains over refined grains is a wise decision for seniors with diabetes. Whole grains, such as quinoa, brown rice, and whole wheat, provide more fiber and nutrients, contributing to better blood sugar management and overall digestive health.

Limiting Added Sugars and Processed Foods: One of the fundamental principles of choosing the right foods involves minimizing the intake of added sugars and highly processed foods. Seniors should be mindful of hidden sugars in packaged products and opt for whole, unprocessed foods whenever possible.

The key to successful food choices lies in balance and variety. Seniors can create enjoyable and satisfying meals by incorporating a diverse range of foods, paying attention to portion sizes, and being mindful of their individual nutritional needs. The goal is not restriction but rather a thoughtful and intentional approach to nourishing the body.

2.1.2 Meal Planning and Portion Control

Meal planning and portion control are integral components of diabetes management, providing seniors with the tools to regulate blood sugar levels and maintain a healthy weight. For seniors, the benefits extend beyond glycemic control; they encompass energy levels, digestion, and overall well-being. Successful meal planning involves a combination of thoughtful preparation, understanding nutritional needs, and mastering portion control strategies.

Balanced Meals: Crafting balanced meals is the cornerstone of effective meal planning. A balanced meal includes a mix of carbohydrates, proteins, and fats, ensuring a steady release of energy and supporting various bodily functions. Seniors should aim for variety, incorporating a range of food groups into each meal.

Consistent Timing: Establishing regular meal times contributes to stable blood sugar levels. Seniors should strive for consistency in the timing of meals and snacks, preventing prolonged periods without nourishment. This practice helps regulate insulin levels and minimizes the risk of blood sugar fluctuations.

Carbohydrate Counting: For seniors with diabetes, understanding the carbohydrate content of foods is a valuable skill. Carbohydrate counting allows for better blood sugar management, as it enables seniors to match insulin doses or oral medications with their carbohydrate intake. Working with a healthcare professional or dietitian can help seniors develop proficiency in carbohydrate counting.

Portion Control Strategies: Seniors often face the challenge of maintaining a healthy weight, and portion control plays a pivotal role in this aspect of diabetes management. Practical strategies for portion control include using smaller plates, measuring serving sizes, and being mindful of portion distortion – the tendency to underestimate the amount of food consumed.

Meal Timing and Physical Activity: Aligning meal timing with physical activity can optimize blood sugar management. Seniors may find it beneficial to plan meals around periods of increased activity, such as after a walk or exercise session. This synchronization helps utilize glucose more efficiently and can contribute to better overall glucose control.

Preparation and Cooking Methods: Seniors can take control of their diet by being involved in meal preparation and choosing cooking methods that enhance nutritional value. Grilling, baking, steaming, and sautéing are healthier alternatives to frying. Preparing meals at home also allows for greater control over ingredients and portion sizes.

Hydration and Mealtime Beverages: Proper hydration is often overlooked in meal planning. Seniors should incorporate water as the primary beverage during meals, avoiding sugary drinks that can contribute to elevated blood sugar levels. Additionally, moderate alcohol consumption, if applicable, should be factored into the overall meal plan.

Individualizing meal plans to meet the specific needs and preferences of seniors is essential for sustained adherence. Seniors are encouraged to experiment with different meal planning approaches, seek support from healthcare professionals or dietitians, and make adjustments based on their unique responses to various foods and strategies.

2.1.3 Managing Sugar and Carbohydrate Intake

Effective management of sugar and carbohydrate intake is a critical aspect of diabetes care for seniors. While carbohydrates are a primary source of energy, understanding how different types of carbohydrates impact blood sugar levels empowers seniors to make informed choices. This section explores strategies for managing sugar and carbohydrate intake, providing practical insights for seniors seeking to maintain glycemic control.

Sugar Awareness: Seniors should develop a keen awareness of hidden sugars in various foods and beverages. Reading food labels can help identify sources of added sugars, allowing seniors to make informed choices and avoid unnecessary spikes in blood sugar levels. Common culprits include sugary drinks, processed snacks, and sweetened cereals.

Natural vs. Added Sugars: Distinguishing between natural sugars found in whole foods and added sugars is crucial for seniors. Whole fruits, for example, contain natural sugars accompanied by fiber and essential nutrients. However, added sugars in processed foods contribute empty calories without nutritional benefits. Seniors are encouraged to prioritize natural sources of sweetness and limit added sugars.

Carbohydrate Quality and Quantity: The quality and quantity of carbohydrates play a significant role in blood sugar management. Seniors should focus on complex carbohydrates with a low glycemic index, such as whole grains, legumes, and non-starchy vegetables. Monitoring portion sizes helps prevent excessive carbohydrate intake and supports stable blood sugar levels.

Meal Timing and Carbohydrates: Distributing carbohydrate intake evenly throughout the day can contribute to better glycemic control. Seniors may find it beneficial to include carbohydrates in each meal and snack, rather than consuming a large amount at one time. This approach helps regulate insulin responses and minimizes post-meal blood sugar spikes.

Carbohydrate Counting and Monitoring: For seniors using insulin or certain medications, carbohydrate counting becomes a valuable skill. It involves estimating the amount of carbohydrates in each meal or snack and adjusting insulin doses accordingly. Regular monitoring of blood sugar levels provides insights into how different foods and meals impact individual responses.

Low-Carb and Mediterranean Approaches: Some seniors may benefit from low-carbohydrate or Mediterranean-style diets, which emphasize whole foods, healthy fats, and lean proteins. These approaches can help manage blood sugar levels, support cardiovascular health, and provide a satisfying and sustainable dietary plan.

Sweeteners and Alternative Choices: Seniors seeking to reduce their sugar intake can explore sugar substitutes and alternative sweeteners. However, it's crucial to use these options in moderation and be mindful of individual responses. Natural sweeteners, such as stevia or monk fruit, may be preferable for some seniors.

Educating seniors about the nuances of sugar and carbohydrate management empowers them to make choices that align with their health goals. The goal is not strict elimination but rather a balanced and individualized approach that fosters enjoyment of food while supporting overall well-being. Regular communication with healthcare professionals or dietitians ensures ongoing guidance and adjustment as needed.

2.2 Regular Exercise for Seniors with Diabetes

The symbiotic relationship between physical activity and diabetes management is particularly pronounced in the senior population. Engaging in regular exercise offers a plethora of benefits, ranging from improved insulin sensitivity to enhanced cardiovascular health. However, seniors must approach exercise with consideration for their unique health circumstances. This section explores the significance of regular exercise for seniors with diabetes and provides insights into safe and effective exercise routines.

Benefits of Exercise for Seniors with Diabetes:

The advantages of regular exercise extend far beyond weight management for seniors with diabetes. Physical activity positively influences various aspects of health, directly impacting diabetes management. Key benefits include:

1. **Improved Insulin Sensitivity:** Regular exercise enhances the body's ability to use insulin effectively, facilitating better blood sugar control. This is

particularly crucial for seniors, as insulin sensitivity tends to decrease with age.

2. **Weight Management:** Maintaining a healthy weight is essential for seniors with diabetes, as excess body weight can contribute to insulin resistance. Regular exercise, when combined with a balanced diet, supports weight management and overall metabolic health.

3. **Cardiovascular Health:** Seniors with diabetes often face an increased risk of cardiovascular complications. Exercise promotes heart health by improving circulation, reducing blood pressure, and lowering the risk of heart disease.

4. **Muscle Strength and Joint Flexibility:** Aging can lead to a decline in muscle mass and joint flexibility. Engaging in strength training exercises helps seniors maintain muscle mass, support joint health, and enhance overall mobility.

5. **Mood and Mental Well-being:** Exercise has proven benefits for mental health, reducing stress, anxiety, and depression. Seniors may find that regular physical activity contributes to a positive outlook and an enhanced sense of well-being.

2.2.1 Safe and Effective Exercises

Ensuring the safety and effectiveness of exercise routines for seniors with diabetes involves a thoughtful and tailored approach. It's essential to consider individual health conditions, physical limitations, and preferences when designing an exercise regimen. Here are some safe and effective exercises for seniors with diabetes:

1. **Walking:** Walking is a low-impact exercise that can be easily incorporated into daily routines. Whether it's a stroll around the neighborhood or a brisk walk in the local park, walking is an excellent cardiovascular activity that promotes blood circulation and supports overall health.

2. **Swimming:** Swimming and water aerobics provide a full-body workout without putting stress on joints. The buoyancy of water reduces impact, making it an ideal exercise for seniors with arthritis or joint issues.

3. **Strength Training:** Building and maintaining muscle mass is crucial for seniors. Strength training exercises, using resistance bands, light weights, or body weight, can help improve muscle strength and joint stability. Focus on major muscle groups, incorporating exercises like squats, lunges, and bicep curls.

4. **Yoga:** Yoga combines physical postures, breathing exercises, and meditation, offering a holistic approach to fitness. Seniors can benefit from improved flexibility, balance, and stress reduction through regular yoga practice.

5. **Tai Chi:** Tai Chi is a gentle and slow-moving exercise that emphasizes balance and coordination. It has been shown to improve mobility, reduce the risk of falls, and enhance overall well-being in seniors.

6. **Stationary Biking:** Stationary bikes provide a low-impact cardiovascular workout. Seniors can adjust the resistance to their comfort level and enjoy the benefits of biking without concerns about balance or joint impact.

7. **Chair Exercises:** For those with limited mobility or difficulty standing, chair exercises offer a seated alternative. These exercises can include leg lifts, seated marches, and arm movements, providing a way to stay active while seated.

Seniors must consult with their healthcare provider before starting a new exercise routine, especially if they have pre-existing health conditions. Additionally, starting slowly and gradually increasing intensity and duration allows the body to adapt and reduces the risk of injury.

2.2.2 Incorporating Physical Activity into Daily Life

For seniors with diabetes, the concept of regular exercise extends beyond structured workout sessions; it involves integrating physical activity into daily life. Small, consistent movements throughout the day contribute to overall health and help manage blood sugar levels. Here are practical ways for seniors to incorporate physical activity into their daily routines:

1. **Morning Stretching Routine:** Starting the day with a gentle stretching routine helps awaken the body, improves flexibility, and sets a positive tone for the day. Seniors can incorporate neck stretches, arm circles, and leg stretches into their morning routine.

2. **Short Walks After Meals:** Taking a short walk after meals can aid in digestion and help regulate blood sugar levels. This doesn't have to be an intense walk; even a ten-minute stroll around the house or garden can make a significant difference.

3. **Gardening:** Gardening is a fulfilling and physically engaging activity. Whether it's planting flowers,

tending to a vegetable garden, or raking leaves, gardening provides a combination of moderate-intensity exercise and the joy of nurturing plants.

4. **Dance:** Seniors can incorporate dance into their routine, whether it's dancing to favorite tunes in the living room or joining a dance class designed for older adults. Dancing not only promotes cardiovascular health but also adds a joyful element to physical activity.

5. **Stair Climbing:** If stairs are accessible, climbing stairs is an effective way to incorporate resistance training into daily life. Seniors can start with a few flights and gradually increase as they build strength.

6. **Seated Exercises:** For those with mobility challenges, seated exercises can be performed while watching television or sitting at a desk. Leg lifts, seated marches, and arm exercises provide a way to stay active in a seated position.

7. **Active Hobbies:** Engaging in hobbies that involve movement, such as painting, woodworking, or playing a musical instrument, can contribute to daily physical activity. Pursuing activities that bring joy while keeping the body active is a win-win.

8. **Family and Social Activities:** Incorporating physical activity into social interactions adds a social dimension to exercise. Seniors can schedule walks with friends, play outdoor games with family, or join community fitness classes.

9. **Technology-Assisted Exercise:** There are various fitness apps and online platforms designed for seniors, offering guided exercises and routines that can be done at home. From chair exercises to gentle yoga sessions, technology provides accessible options for staying active.

10. **Balancing Exercises:** Improving balance is crucial for seniors to prevent falls. Simple balancing exercises, such as standing on one leg while brushing teeth or doing heel-to-toe walks, can be seamlessly integrated into daily routines.

The key to the successful integration of physical activity into daily life is finding activities that are enjoyable and sustainable. Seniors are encouraged to explore different options, listen to their bodies, and make adjustments based on individual comfort levels. Regular communication with healthcare providers ensures that the chosen activities align with overall health goals and existing medical conditions.

Regular exercise is a potent tool for seniors managing diabetes, offering a multitude of physical and mental health benefits. By understanding safe and effective exercises and incorporating physical activity into daily life, seniors can take proactive steps toward optimal diabetes management, improved overall well-being, and a fulfilling and active lifestyle.

2.3 Stress Management and Sleep

For seniors navigating the challenges of diabetes, stress management and quality sleep are integral components of a holistic approach to well-being. The intricate interplay between stress, sleep, and diabetes requires careful consideration, as disruptions in these areas can significantly impact blood sugar levels and overall health. This section explores the profound impact of stress on blood sugar levels and provides practical strategies for relaxation and achieving restorative sleep.

2.3.1 Impact of Stress on Blood Sugar Levels

Stress, whether acute or chronic, triggers a cascade of physiological responses that can profoundly influence blood sugar levels. Seniors with diabetes need to be particularly attuned to the impact of stress, as it can contribute to fluctuations in glucose levels and complicate diabetes management. Understanding the connection between stress and blood sugar is the first step in developing effective stress management strategies.

Stress Hormones and Blood Sugar: When the body perceives a stressor, the "fight or flight" response is activated, leading to the release of stress hormones such as cortisol and adrenaline. These hormones trigger the liver to release stored glucose into the bloodstream, providing a quick source of energy for the perceived threat. While this response is essential for survival in acute situations, chronic stress can lead to sustained elevated blood sugar levels.

Insulin Resistance and Inflammation: Prolonged stress is associated with insulin resistance, where the body's cells become less responsive to insulin's effects. This can lead to an increase in blood sugar levels, as insulin is less effective in facilitating glucose uptake by cells. Additionally, chronic stress promotes inflammation, further contributing to insulin resistance and disrupting normal blood sugar regulation.

Emotional Eating and Food Choices: Stress can influence eating behaviors, leading to emotional eating or cravings for high-calorie, sugary foods. Seniors with diabetes may find themselves reaching for comfort foods during times of stress, which can contribute to blood sugar spikes. Understanding and addressing these patterns is crucial for maintaining glycemic control.

Impact on Lifestyle Habits: Chronic stress can also affect lifestyle habits that are essential for diabetes management. Seniors may experience disruptions in sleep, reduced motivation for physical activity, and difficulty adhering to a healthy diet. These factors collectively contribute to challenges in blood sugar control.

Strategies for Managing Stress:

Recognizing the impact of stress on blood sugar levels underscores the importance of implementing effective stress management strategies. Seniors with diabetes can benefit from incorporating the following approaches into their daily lives:

1. **Mindfulness and Meditation:** Mindfulness practices, such as meditation and deep breathing exercises, promote relaxation and help mitigate the physiological effects of stress. Seniors can dedicate a few minutes each day to mindfulness, fostering a sense of calm and reducing stress hormone levels.

2. **Physical Activity:** Regular physical activity is not only beneficial for blood sugar control but also acts as a powerful stress reducer. Seniors can explore activities like walking, yoga, or tai chi, which combine movement with mindfulness, enhancing both physical and mental well-being.

3. **Social Support:** Maintaining social connections is crucial for managing stress. Seniors can seek support from family, friends, or support groups, providing opportunities for sharing experiences, receiving encouragement, and fostering a sense of community.

4. **Time Management:** Efficient time management can alleviate the stress associated with overwhelming tasks. Seniors can create realistic schedules, prioritize tasks, and break larger goals into smaller, more manageable steps.

5. **Hobbies and Leisure Activities:** Engaging in hobbies and leisure activities provides a welcome distraction from stressors. Whether it's reading, gardening, or pursuing creative outlets, seniors can find joy and relaxation in activities that bring them fulfillment.

6. **Counseling and Therapy:** Professional counseling or therapy can offer valuable tools for coping with stress. Seniors may explore cognitive-behavioral therapy (CBT) or other therapeutic approaches to address stressors and develop effective coping strategies.

7. **Relaxation Techniques:** Incorporating relaxation techniques, such as progressive muscle relaxation or guided imagery, can promote a sense of calm and

relaxation. These techniques can be beneficial before bedtime to improve sleep quality.

Quality sleep is a cornerstone of overall health, and for seniors managing diabetes, it plays a pivotal role in glycemic control. Sleep disturbances can exacerbate insulin resistance and contribute to heightened stress levels. This section explores the impact of sleep on diabetes and provides practical strategies for seniors to enhance relaxation and achieve restorative sleep.

The Bidirectional Relationship: The relationship between diabetes and sleep is bidirectional, meaning each condition can influence the other. Poorly managed diabetes can contribute to sleep disturbances, while insufficient or disrupted sleep can adversely affect blood sugar control. Understanding this interplay is crucial for seniors seeking comprehensive diabetes care.

Impact of Sleep on Blood Sugar Levels: Inadequate or poor-quality sleep can lead to insulin resistance, and impaired glucose metabolism, and contribute to elevated blood sugar levels. Seniors may experience the dawn phenomenon, where blood sugar levels rise in the early morning due to a surge in cortisol. Quality sleep is essential for mitigating these effects and promoting optimal glycemic control.

Sleep Disorders and Diabetes: Seniors with diabetes may be at an increased risk of certain sleep disorders, such as sleep apnea. Sleep apnea is characterized by pauses in breathing during sleep, leading to fragmented sleep and decreased oxygen levels. This condition can exacerbate insulin resistance and contribute to daytime fatigue.

Circadian Rhythms and Diabetes: The body's internal clock, known as the circadian rhythm, plays a crucial role in regulating various physiological processes, including glucose metabolism. Disruptions to circadian rhythms, such as irregular sleep patterns or shift work, can negatively impact blood sugar control.

Strategies for Improving Sleep Quality:

Recognizing the importance of quality sleep in diabetes management prompts the exploration of strategies to enhance sleep hygiene and promote restorative sleep for seniors:

1. **Consistent Sleep Schedule:** Seniors should aim for a consistent sleep schedule, going to bed and waking up at the same time each day. This helps regulate the body's internal clock and promotes the establishment of a healthy sleep-wake cycle.

2. **Create a Relaxing Bedtime Routine:** Establishing a calming bedtime routine signals to the body that it's time to wind down. This can include activities such as reading, gentle stretching, or listening to soothing music. Avoiding stimulating activities or electronic devices before bedtime is crucial for a tranquil transition to sleep.

3. **Optimize Sleep Environment:** Creating a comfortable and conducive sleep environment is essential. Seniors should ensure their bedroom is dark, quiet, and cool. Investing in a comfortable mattress and pillows can also contribute to a more restful sleep.

4. **Limit Stimulants and Heavy Meals:** Seniors should be mindful of stimulants such as caffeine and nicotine, especially in the hours leading up to bedtime. Additionally, heavy or spicy meals close to bedtime may contribute to indigestion, disrupting sleep. Opting for a light snack if needed is a preferable choice.

5. **Regular Physical Activity:** Engaging in regular physical activity supports overall health and can contribute to better sleep quality. However, seniors should avoid vigorous exercise close to bedtime, opting for gentler activities such as stretching or relaxation exercises.

6. **Manage Stress Before Bed:** Implementing stress management techniques before bedtime can help seniors unwind and prepare for a restful night. This can include mindfulness practices, deep breathing exercises, or gentle yoga stretches.

7. **Limit Screen Time:** The blue light emitted by screens can interfere with the production of the sleep hormone melatonin. Seniors should limit screen time to the hour before bedtime and consider using "night mode" settings on devices.

8. **Address Sleep Disorders:** Seniors experiencing persistent sleep disturbances or symptoms of sleep disorders, such as sleep apnea, should seek evaluation and treatment. Addressing underlying sleep issues is crucial for improving overall health and diabetes management.

9. **Limit Naps:** While short daytime naps can be beneficial, excessively long or irregular napping patterns can interfere with nighttime sleep. Seniors

should aim for brief, rejuvenating naps earlier in the day if needed.

10. **Hydration and Medication Management:** Proper hydration is essential, but seniors should be mindful of excessive fluid intake close to bedtime to avoid disruptions due to bathroom visits. Additionally, adherence to medication schedules, including diabetes medications, is crucial for maintaining stability in blood sugar levels during sleep.

By prioritizing relaxation and quality sleep, seniors with diabetes can enhance their overall health and empower themselves in the management of their condition. Implementing a holistic approach that includes stress management and sleep hygiene contributes to a comprehensive and sustainable strategy for diabetes care. Regular communication with healthcare providers ensures that these lifestyle changes align with individual health goals and medical considerations.

Recognizing the intricate connections between stress, sleep, and diabetes management is essential for seniors navigating the complexities of living with diabetes. By incorporating effective stress management strategies and prioritizing quality sleep, seniors can take proactive steps toward achieving optimal glycemic control and fostering overall well-being.

Chapter 3:

Medications and Insulin Management

Effectively managing diabetes in seniors often involves a combination of lifestyle changes and medications. In this chapter, we delve into the diverse landscape of diabetes medications, providing an overview of commonly prescribed drugs and insulin management strategies tailored to the unique needs of seniors.

3.1 Overview of Diabetes Medications for Seniors

Diabetes management in seniors is a nuanced journey that may necessitate the inclusion of medications to achieve optimal blood sugar control. A comprehensive understanding of the available medications is essential for both seniors and their healthcare providers. This section provides an overview of diabetes medications for seniors, encompassing both oral and injectable options.

3.1.1 Oral Medications

Oral medications are a common component of diabetes management, often prescribed to seniors to enhance insulin sensitivity, reduce glucose production by the liver, and improve overall blood sugar control. Understanding the different classes of oral medications is crucial for tailoring treatment plans to individual needs.

Biguanides: Metformin is a widely prescribed biguanide medication that is often the first-line oral treatment for type 2 diabetes in seniors. It works by reducing glucose production in the liver and improving insulin sensitivity in peripheral tissues. Metformin is known for its safety profile, making it a suitable option for many seniors. However, it is important to monitor kidney function, as metformin can affect renal health.

Sulfonylureas: Sulfonylureas stimulate the pancreas to release more insulin. While they can be effective in lowering blood sugar levels, they may pose a risk of hypoglycemia (low blood sugar) in seniors. Common sulfonylureas include glyburide, glipizide, and glimepiride. Careful consideration of individual health status and the risk of hypoglycemia is essential when prescribing sulfonylureas to seniors.

Dipeptidyl Peptidase-4 (DPP-4) Inhibitors: DPP-4 inhibitors, such as sitagliptin and saxagliptin, work by increasing insulin release and decreasing glucagon secretion. They are oral medications that are generally well-tolerated and have a lower risk of hypoglycemia compared to some other classes. Seniors may benefit from DPP-4 inhibitors due to their ease of use and favorable side effect profile.

Thiazolidinediones (TZDs): TZDs, including pioglitazone and rosiglitazone, improve insulin sensitivity in peripheral tissues. While effective in managing blood sugar levels, TZDs have been associated with side effects such as fluid retention and an increased risk of fractures. Careful consideration of individual health conditions, including heart and bone health, is important when prescribing TZDs to seniors.

Alpha-Glucosidase Inhibitors: These medications, including acarbose and miglitol, slow down the absorption of carbohydrates in the digestive tract. While they can help control post-meal blood sugar spikes, they may also cause gastrointestinal side effects. Seniors need to be aware of potential digestive issues and work closely with healthcare providers to adjust dosage if necessary.

Sodium-Glucose Cotransporter-2 (SGLT-2) Inhibitors: SGLT-2 inhibitors, such as canagliflozin and empagliflozin, work by reducing glucose reabsorption in the kidneys, leading to increased excretion of glucose in the urine. These medications have shown cardiovascular and kidney benefits. However, seniors should be cautious of potential side effects such as urinary tract infections and dehydration.

Understanding the mechanisms of action, potential side effects, and individual considerations for each class of oral medication is crucial for tailoring treatment plans to the specific needs and health status of seniors with diabetes.

3.1.2 Injectable Medications

In some cases, seniors may require injectable medications to manage their diabetes effectively. Injectable medications encompass both non-insulin injectables and insulin, offering additional options for blood sugar control.

Non-Insulin Injectable Medications:

Glucagon-like Peptide-1 (GLP-1) Receptor Agonists: GLP-1 receptor agonists, such as exenatide and liraglutide, mimic the action of the incretin hormone GLP-1. They stimulate insulin release, reduce glucagon secretion, and slow down gastric emptying. GLP-1 agonists are administered via injection and can be beneficial for seniors seeking weight loss, as they are associated with appetite reduction. However, seniors need to be aware of potential gastrointestinal side effects.

Amylin Analogs: Pramlintide is an amylin analog that mimics the action of the hormone amylin, which is deficient in individuals with diabetes. It helps regulate blood sugar levels by slowing down gastric emptying and reducing post-meal blood sugar spikes. Pramlintide is administered before meals via injection and can be considered for seniors who need additional blood sugar control.

Understanding the role and administration of non-insulin injectable medications provides seniors and their healthcare providers with additional options for personalized diabetes management.

Insulin Management:

For some seniors with diabetes, insulin therapy may be necessary to achieve optimal blood sugar control. Insulin is a hormone that helps regulate blood sugar by facilitating the uptake of glucose into cells. There are different types of insulin, classified based on their onset, peak, and duration of action.

Rapid-Acting Insulin: Rapid-acting insulin, such as insulin lispro and insulin aspart, has a quick onset and is taken just before or with meals to manage post-meal blood sugar spikes. This type of insulin is beneficial for seniors who need precise control over their blood sugar levels during meals.

Short-Acting Insulin: Short-acting insulin, such as regular insulin, has a slightly slower onset compared to rapid-acting insulin. It is typically taken around 30 minutes before meals to manage blood sugar levels during the meal. Seniors using short-acting insulin need to coordinate their injections with their mealtime.

Intermediate-Acting Insulin: Intermediate-acting insulin, such as NPH insulin, has a more prolonged duration of action compared to rapid or short-acting insulin. It is often used to provide basal insulin coverage between meals and overnight. This type of insulin can be beneficial for seniors who require a steady level of insulin throughout the day and night.

Long-Acting Insulin: Long-acting insulin, such as insulin glargine and insulin detemir, provides a continuous, basal level of insulin over an extended period. It is typically taken once or twice a day to maintain a baseline level of insulin between meals and overnight. Long-acting insulin is suitable for seniors seeking a consistent and predictable insulin regimen.

Premixed Insulin: Premixed insulin combines a specific ratio of rapid-acting or short-acting insulin with intermediate-acting insulin. It provides both mealtime and basal insulin coverage in a single injection. Premixed insulin can be convenient for seniors who prefer a simpler insulin regimen.

Seniors and their healthcare providers need to collaborate closely in determining the most appropriate insulin regimen based on individual needs, lifestyle, and health status. Regular monitoring of blood sugar levels and adjustments to insulin dosages may be necessary to achieve and maintain optimal glycemic control.

The management of diabetes in seniors encompasses a diverse array of medications, ranging from oral medications to injectable options, including both non-insulin injectables and insulin. Tailoring treatment plans to the unique needs of seniors involves a thorough understanding of the mechanisms of action, potential side effects, and individual considerations for each medication class. The collaboration between seniors and their healthcare providers is paramount in achieving optimal blood sugar control and enhancing overall well-being.

3.2 Insulin Therapy

Insulin therapy is a cornerstone in the management of diabetes, providing a targeted approach to regulate blood sugar levels. For seniors with diabetes, insulin therapy can be a crucial component of their treatment plan, addressing individual needs and achieving optimal glycemic control.

3.2.1 Types of Insulin

Understanding the different types of insulin is fundamental for tailoring insulin therapy to the specific requirements of seniors. Insulin is categorized based on its onset, peak, and duration of action, allowing for a personalized approach to blood sugar management.

Rapid-Acting Insulin: Rapid-acting insulin is characterized by its quick onset and short duration of action. It is designed to address post-meal spikes in blood sugar levels. Common rapid-acting insulins include insulin lispro, insulin aspart, and insulin glulisine. Seniors may administer rapid-acting insulin just before or with meals to manage the increase in blood sugar that occurs after eating.

Short-Acting Insulin: Short-acting insulin, often referred to as regular insulin, has a slightly slower onset compared to rapid-acting insulin. It is typically taken about 30 minutes before meals to manage blood sugar levels during the meal. Regular insulin provides a more extended coverage compared to rapid-acting insulin and is suitable for seniors who require a pre-meal injection to support mealtime blood sugar control.

Intermediate-Acting Insulin: Intermediate-acting insulin, such as NPH (Neutral Protamine Hagedorn) insulin, has a more prolonged duration of action compared to rapid or short-acting insulin. It provides a basal level of insulin coverage between meals and overnight. NPH insulin is often used to address the fasting and overnight periods when blood sugar levels may rise. It can be beneficial for seniors seeking more extended coverage to maintain stable blood sugar levels.

Long-Acting Insulin: Long-acting insulin provides a continuous, basal level of insulin over an extended period. It is designed to maintain a baseline level of insulin between meals and overnight. Common long-acting insulins include insulin glargine and insulin detemir. These insulins offer a more consistent and predictable insulin release, providing foundational support for blood sugar control throughout the day and night.

Premixed Insulin: Premixed insulin combines a specific ratio of rapid-acting or short-acting insulin with intermediate-acting insulin. This combination provides both mealtime and basal insulin coverage in a single injection. Premixed insulin can be convenient for seniors who prefer a simplified insulin regimen, offering the benefits of both rapid-acting and intermediate-acting insulins in one injection.

Choosing the most appropriate type of insulin involves considering individual lifestyle, meal patterns, and preferences. Seniors and their healthcare providers collaborate to create a personalized insulin regimen that aligns with the senior's unique needs and facilitates optimal blood sugar control.

3.2.2 Insulin Injection Techniques

Effective insulin therapy requires proper injection techniques to ensure accurate dosage delivery and minimize the risk of complications. Seniors need to be familiar with various injection methods and choose the technique that suits their comfort level and individual circumstances.

Subcutaneous Injection: Subcutaneous injection is the most common method for administering insulin. Seniors typically inject insulin into the fatty tissue just beneath the skin. The abdomen is a commonly chosen site due to its easy accessibility. Other suitable areas include the thighs, buttocks, and upper arms. Rotating injection sites helps prevent the development of lumps or fatty deposits at the injection site.

Insulin Pens: Insulin pens are user-friendly devices that simplify the injection process. They consist of a cartridge of insulin and a disposable needle. Seniors can dial the desired dose on the pen and inject the insulin by pressing a button. Insulin pens are convenient and often come preloaded with insulin, reducing the need for drawing insulin from vials.

Insulin Syringes: Traditional insulin syringes consist of a needle attached to a syringe, allowing seniors to draw insulin from vials and inject the desired dosage. While syringes may require additional steps, some seniors may prefer the control and flexibility they offer.

Injection Angle and Depth: The angle and depth of the injection play a role in ensuring proper insulin absorption. Subcutaneous injections are typically administered at a 90-degree angle, ensuring that the insulin is delivered into the fatty tissue beneath the skin. Seniors can pinch the skin before injecting to create a small fold, providing a suitable area for injection.

Needle Length: The choice of needle length depends on factors such as body mass and injection site. Shorter needles may be suitable for seniors with less subcutaneous tissue, while longer needles may be appropriate for those with more fatty tissue. Healthcare providers can guide seniors in selecting the most suitable needle length for their insulin injections.

Proper Disposal of Needles: Seniors must be diligent in the safe disposal of needles and syringes. Sharps containers or puncture-resistant containers are recommended for the disposal of used needles. This practice ensures the prevention of accidental needlestick injuries and promotes environmental safety.

Mastering insulin injection techniques empowers seniors to take an active role in their diabetes management. Regular communication with healthcare providers ensures ongoing support, guidance, and adjustments as needed.

3.2.3 Monitoring and Adjusting Insulin Dosages

Achieving optimal blood sugar control with insulin therapy involves regular monitoring of blood glucose levels and making adjustments to insulin dosages as necessary. Seniors, in collaboration with their healthcare providers, play an active role in this ongoing process.

Self-Monitoring of Blood Glucose (SMBG): Self-monitoring of blood glucose is a vital aspect of insulin therapy for seniors. Regular blood glucose monitoring allows seniors to track their blood sugar levels and identify patterns or trends. Portable glucose meters provide a convenient means for seniors to check their blood sugar levels at home or on the go. The frequency of blood glucose monitoring may vary based on individual treatment plans and healthcare provider recommendations.

Target Blood Sugar Levels: Setting target blood sugar levels is a collaborative effort between seniors and their healthcare providers. Target ranges are personalized based on factors such as age, overall health, and individual treatment goals. Seniors should be aware of their target ranges for fasting and post-meal blood sugar levels, allowing them to gauge the effectiveness of their insulin therapy.

Adjusting Insulin Dosages: The adjustment of insulin dosages is a dynamic process that requires regular communication between seniors and healthcare providers. Factors such as changes in diet, physical activity, illness, or medications may necessitate modifications to insulin dosages. Seniors should be vigilant in reporting any changes in their routine or health status to their healthcare team.

Hypoglycemia Management: Seniors on insulin therapy need to be knowledgeable about hypoglycemia (low blood sugar) symptoms and management. Hypoglycemia can occur when insulin doses are too high, or there are variations in meal timing and composition. Seniors should have a plan in place for treating hypoglycemia, which may include consuming a fast-acting carbohydrate, such as glucose tablets or juice.

Hyperglycemia Recognition and Response: Similarly, recognizing the symptoms of hyperglycemia (high blood sugar) is essential. Seniors should be aware of signs such as excessive thirst, frequent urination, and fatigue. If hyperglycemia is detected, healthcare providers may recommend adjustments to insulin dosages or other aspects of the treatment plan.

Regular Healthcare Visits: Regular healthcare visits are crucial for seniors on insulin therapy. These visits provide opportunities for healthcare providers to review blood sugar data, assess overall health, and make necessary adjustments to insulin regimens. Seniors should actively participate in these discussions, sharing their experiences, concerns, and any challenges they may be facing.

Insulin therapy is a dynamic and personalized aspect of diabetes management for seniors. Understanding the different types of insulin, mastering injection techniques, and actively participating in monitoring and adjusting insulin dosages empower seniors to take control of their diabetes. Collaboration with healthcare providers ensures a tailored approach that aligns with individual needs and promotes optimal blood sugar control, contributing to overall well-being.

Chapter 4:

Monitoring Blood Sugar Levels

Effective monitoring of blood sugar levels is a fundamental aspect of diabetes management for seniors. This chapter explores the importance of regular monitoring, the tools available, such as blood glucose meters and continuous glucose monitoring (CGM), and the establishment of target blood sugar ranges tailored to the unique needs of seniors.

4.1 Importance of Regular Monitoring

For seniors living with diabetes, regular monitoring of blood sugar levels is a cornerstone of effective self-management. This process provides valuable insights into the impact of various factors on blood sugar levels, allowing seniors and their healthcare providers to make informed decisions about treatment plans, lifestyle adjustments, and overall well-being.

4.1.1 Blood Glucose Meters and Continuous Glucose Monitoring (CGM)

Blood glucose meters and continuous glucose monitoring (CGM) systems are essential tools that enable seniors to monitor their blood sugar levels accurately and consistently. These technologies empower seniors to take an active role in their diabetes management, providing real-time information that guides decision-making.

Blood Glucose Meters: Blood glucose meters, also known as glucometers, are handheld devices that measure blood sugar levels from a small drop of blood. Seniors can obtain a blood sample by pricking their fingertips with a lancet and then placing the blood on a test strip, which is inserted into the meter. The meter then displays the current blood sugar level.

Advantages of Blood Glucose Meters:

- **Portability:** Blood glucose meters are compact and portable, allowing seniors to monitor their blood sugar levels at home, work, or while traveling.

- **Affordability:** Compared to some continuous monitoring options, blood glucose meters are often more affordable, making them accessible to a broad range of seniors.

- **User-Friendly:** Blood glucose meters are user-friendly, with simple interfaces and easy-to-follow instructions for obtaining and interpreting blood sugar readings.

Considerations for Seniors:

- **Consistent Testing Routine:** Seniors benefit from establishing a consistent routine for blood sugar testing, such as testing before meals, after meals, and at bedtime.

- **Record Keeping:** Keeping a log or using digital apps to record blood sugar readings, along with additional notes about meals, physical activity, and medication, provides a comprehensive overview for both seniors and healthcare providers.

Continuous Glucose Monitoring (CGM): Continuous glucose monitoring (CGM) systems offer a dynamic and continuous view of blood sugar trends throughout the day and night. These systems consist of a tiny sensor inserted under the skin that measures glucose levels in the interstitial fluid. The sensor communicates with a transmitter, which wirelessly sends data to a receiver or a smartphone app.

Advantages of CGM Systems:

- **Real-Time Data:** CGM systems provide real-time data, allowing seniors to monitor their blood sugar levels continuously without the need for frequent fingerstick tests.

- **Trend Analysis:** CGM systems offer trend analysis, illustrating how blood sugar levels change over time. This information helps seniors and healthcare providers identify patterns and make timely adjustments to treatment plans.

- **Alerts and Alarms:** CGM systems can be programmed to provide alerts and alarms when blood sugar levels are approaching high or low thresholds, enhancing proactive management.

Considerations for Seniors:

- **Sensor Placement:** Seniors should follow guidelines for sensor placement, choosing areas with sufficient subcutaneous tissue for accurate readings. Rotating sensor sites helps prevent skin irritation.

- **Device Integration:** Some CGM systems integrate with insulin pumps or smartphones, streamlining data access and enhancing overall convenience.

- **Insurance Coverage:** Seniors should check with their insurance providers to determine coverage for CGM systems, as these technologies may be covered under certain plans.

4.1.2 Target Blood Sugar Ranges

Establishing target blood sugar ranges is a collaborative effort between seniors and their healthcare providers. These targets guide self-monitoring practices, treatment decisions, and lifestyle adjustments, aiming to achieve optimal blood sugar control while minimizing the risk of complications.

Fasting Blood Sugar Targets: Fasting blood sugar levels, measured in the morning before eating or drinking anything except water, provide insight into overnight glucose control. Target ranges for fasting blood sugar may vary based on individual factors such as age, overall health, and specific treatment goals.

Postprandial Blood Sugar Targets: Postprandial blood sugar levels, measured after meals, offer information about how the body processes and responds to food. Seniors may target specific ranges after meals to prevent post-meal spikes in blood sugar.

HbA1c Targets: Hemoglobin A1c (HbA1c) is a measure of average blood sugar levels over the past two to three months. Seniors and their healthcare providers set target HbA1c levels based on individual health status, aiming for values that reflect good long-term blood sugar control.

Individualization of Targets: The establishment of target blood sugar ranges considers individual factors such as age, overall health, coexisting medical conditions, and the presence of complications. Seniors with diabetes should work closely with their healthcare providers to determine personalized targets that align with their unique circumstances.

Factors Influencing Blood Sugar Targets: Several factors can influence target blood sugar ranges for seniors, and adjustments may be necessary based on individual considerations:

- **Age:** Blood sugar targets may be adjusted for seniors to accommodate changes in metabolism and overall health.

- **Health Status:** Coexisting medical conditions, such as cardiovascular disease or kidney issues, can impact target ranges.

- **Complications:** The presence of diabetes-related complications, such as neuropathy or retinopathy, may influence target levels.

- **Medications:** The type and dosage of diabetes medications, including insulin, can affect blood sugar targets.

Regular Review and Adjustments: Target blood sugar ranges are not static and may need to be adjusted over time. Regular reviews with healthcare providers, along with ongoing communication about lifestyle changes, medication adjustments, and overall health, ensure that target ranges remain relevant and effective.

The importance of regular blood sugar monitoring cannot be overstated for seniors living with diabetes. Whether utilizing blood glucose meters or continuous glucose monitoring systems, seniors gain valuable insights into their blood sugar trends, enabling informed decision-making and proactive management. Establishing target blood sugar ranges, personalized to individual circumstances, serves as a guiding framework for optimal diabetes control and overall well-being.

Ongoing collaboration with healthcare providers ensures that monitoring practices and target ranges remain tailored to the unique needs of seniors with diabetes.

4.2 Recognizing and Managing Hypoglycemia

Hypoglycemia, or low blood sugar, is a common concern for seniors with diabetes. Recognizing the symptoms and understanding the causes of hypoglycemia is essential for proactive management and prompt intervention. This section explores the intricacies of hypoglycemia, offering insights into its symptoms, underlying causes, and effective emergency responses for seniors.

4.2.1 Symptoms and Causes

Symptoms of Hypoglycemia:

Seniors need to be vigilant about recognizing the symptoms of hypoglycemia, as prompt intervention is crucial to prevent complications. The symptoms of hypoglycemia can vary among individuals, but common signs include:

1. **Shakiness or Trembling:** Seniors may experience trembling or shakiness, often noticeable in the hands or other parts of the body.

2. **Sweating:** Profuse sweating, even in cool or comfortable temperatures, can be a symptom of hypoglycemia.

3. **Irritability or Mood Changes:** Seniors may become irritable, anxious, or experience sudden mood swings.

4. **Dizziness or Lightheadedness:** Feeling dizzy or lightheaded is a common symptom of low blood sugar.

5. **Confusion:** Seniors may become confused or have difficulty concentrating.

6. **Weakness or Fatigue:** Hypoglycemia can lead to a sudden feeling of weakness or fatigue.

7. **Blurred Vision:** Vision changes, such as blurred or double vision, may occur during episodes of low blood sugar.

8. **Headache:** Seniors may experience headaches as a result of hypoglycemia.

9. **Hunger:** A sudden and intense feeling of hunger can be a signal of low blood sugar.

10. **Nausea or Upset Stomach:** Hypoglycemia may cause nausea or an upset stomach in some seniors.

It's important to note that individual responses to hypoglycemia can vary, and seniors may not experience all of these symptoms. Recognizing even one or two of these signs should prompt seniors to check their blood sugar levels and take appropriate action.

Causes of Hypoglycemia:

Understanding the causes of hypoglycemia is vital for seniors to prevent and manage low blood sugar effectively. Common causes include:

1. **Medication Mismatch:** Seniors on diabetes medications, especially insulin or sulfonylureas, may experience hypoglycemia if the dosage is too high or if there is a mismatch between medication, food intake, and physical activity.

2. **Delay or Missed Meals:** Skipping meals or delaying meals can lead to drops in blood sugar levels, particularly for seniors taking diabetes medications.

3. **Inadequate Carbohydrate Intake:** A diet lacking sufficient carbohydrates can contribute to hypoglycemia. Seniors should ensure a balanced intake of carbohydrates as part of their meal planning.

4. **Increased Physical Activity:** Engaging in more physical activity than usual without adjusting diabetes medications or carbohydrate intake can lead to hypoglycemia.

5. **Alcohol Consumption:** Drinking alcohol, especially on an empty stomach, can increase the risk of hypoglycemia. Seniors should consume alcohol in moderation and ideally with food.

6. **Medical Conditions:** Certain medical conditions, such as kidney or liver disease, can affect the metabolism of medications and contribute to hypoglycemia.

7. **Insulinoma:** In rare cases, a tumor in the pancreas called an insulinoma can lead to excessive insulin production, causing hypoglycemia. However, this is uncommon.

Seniors and their healthcare providers should work collaboratively to identify specific factors contributing to hypoglycemia in individual cases. Adjustments to medications, meal plans, and lifestyle can help manage and prevent episodes of low blood sugar.

Responding promptly to hypoglycemia is crucial to prevent complications and ensure the well-being of seniors with diabetes. The following steps outline an effective emergency response:

1. Check Blood Sugar Levels:

- Seniors should check their blood sugar levels using a blood glucose meter or continuous glucose monitoring (CGM) system to confirm if hypoglycemia is the cause of symptoms.

2. Consume Rapid-Acting Carbohydrates:

- Seniors should have a readily available source of rapid-acting carbohydrates, such as glucose tablets, gel, or a small serving of fruit juice or regular soda. Consuming these carbohydrates helps raise blood sugar levels quickly.

3. Follow the 15-15 Rule:

- The 15-15 rule is a commonly recommended approach to treating hypoglycemia. Seniors should consume 15 grams of rapidly absorbed carbohydrates, wait for 15 minutes, and then recheck their blood sugar levels. If blood sugar remains low, an additional 15 grams of carbohydrates may be needed.

4. Include Protein or Complex Carbohydrates:

- After the initial treatment with rapid-acting carbohydrates, seniors should include a source of protein or complex carbohydrates to sustain blood sugar levels and prevent a subsequent drop.

5. Seek Medical Attention if Necessary:

- If symptoms persist, or worsen, or if the senior is unable to consume oral carbohydrates, emergency medical assistance should be sought. In severe cases, the administration of glucagon may be necessary, and seniors and their caregivers should be trained on its use.

6. Inform Others:

- Seniors living alone should inform family members, neighbors, or caregivers about their condition and the necessary steps to take in case of a hypoglycemic episode. Wearing a medical alert bracelet or necklace indicating diabetes can also be beneficial.

7. Reflect on Contributing Factors:

- After managing the immediate episode of hypoglycemia, seniors should reflect on potential contributing factors. This may involve reviewing recent meals, physical activity, and medication dosages. Adjustments may be needed to prevent future occurrences.

It's essential for seniors to have an emergency plan in place and to communicate this plan with those around them. Being proactive in managing hypoglycemia and seeking prompt medical attention when needed can contribute to the overall safety and well-being of seniors with diabetes.

In conclusion, recognizing and managing hypoglycemia is a critical aspect of diabetes care for seniors. By being aware of the symptoms, understanding the potential causes, and having an effective emergency response plan in place, seniors can navigate episodes of low blood sugar with confidence. Collaboration with healthcare providers, regular monitoring of blood sugar levels, and adjustments to medications and lifestyle contribute to proactive hypoglycemia management, empowering seniors to live well with diabetes.

Chapter 5:

Preventing and Managing Complications

Diabetes, when left unmanaged, can lead to various complications affecting different organ systems. This chapter focuses on preventing and managing complications in seniors with diabetes, with a specific emphasis on cardiovascular health. Understanding the impact of diabetes on the heart and adopting lifestyle strategies for heart health are pivotal aspects of comprehensive diabetes care for seniors.

5.1 Cardiovascular Health for Seniors with Diabetes

Cardiovascular health is of paramount importance for seniors with diabetes. Diabetes can significantly impact the heart and blood vessels, increasing the risk of cardiovascular complications. This section explores the intricate connection between diabetes and cardiovascular health, shedding light on the implications and offering practical lifestyle strategies to promote heart health among seniors.

5.1.1 Impact of Diabetes on the Heart

Seniors with diabetes face an elevated risk of cardiovascular complications due to the intricate interplay between diabetes and the cardiovascular system. Understanding these dynamics is crucial for proactive management and preventive measures.

Atherosclerosis and Coronary Artery Disease (CAD): One of the primary cardiovascular complications associated with diabetes is atherosclerosis, a condition characterized by the buildup of plaque in the arteries. Diabetes accelerates the progression of atherosclerosis, particularly in the coronary arteries, leading to coronary artery disease (CAD). Seniors with diabetes have a higher likelihood of developing narrowed or blocked coronary arteries, impeding blood flow to the heart muscle and increasing the risk of heart attacks.

Hypertension (High Blood Pressure): Diabetes and hypertension often coexist, forming a dangerous combination that significantly raises the risk of cardiovascular events. Diabetes can contribute to the development and worsening of hypertension, putting additional strain on the heart and blood vessels. Seniors with diabetes should monitor and manage their blood pressure closely to reduce the risk of complications.

Myocardial Infarction (Heart Attack): The increased prevalence of atherosclerosis and the greater likelihood of hypertension in seniors with diabetes heighten the risk of myocardial infarction, commonly known as a heart attack. Seniors should be vigilant about recognizing the signs of a heart attack, including chest pain or discomfort, shortness of breath, and pain or discomfort in the arms, back, neck, jaw, or stomach.

Heart Failure: Diabetes is a significant risk factor for heart failure, a condition where the heart is unable to pump blood effectively. The combination of atherosclerosis, hypertension, and other factors associated with diabetes can compromise the heart's ability to function optimally. Seniors with diabetes should be aware of the symptoms of heart failure, such as fatigue, swelling in the legs and abdomen, and difficulty breathing.

Arrhythmias: Diabetes can contribute to the development of arrhythmias, and irregular heartbeats that may disrupt the normal rhythm of the heart. Seniors with diabetes should be mindful of symptoms such as palpitations, dizziness, and fainting, which may indicate the presence of arrhythmias.

Diabetes has far-reaching effects on cardiovascular health, necessitating a comprehensive approach to minimize the risk of complications. Seniors, along with their healthcare providers, play a pivotal role in managing diabetes to protect their heart health.

5.1.2 Lifestyle Strategies for Heart Health

Promoting heart health involves a combination of lifestyle modifications, regular monitoring, and collaborative efforts between seniors and their healthcare providers. Implementing the following strategies can significantly contribute to the prevention and management of cardiovascular complications in seniors with diabetes.

Healthy Eating Habits: A heart-healthy diet is a cornerstone of diabetes management and cardiovascular health. Seniors should focus on:

- **Balanced Nutrient Intake:** Consuming a well-balanced diet that includes a variety of fruits, vegetables, whole grains, lean proteins, and healthy fats supports overall health and helps manage blood sugar levels.

- **Limiting Sodium Intake:** Seniors should be mindful of their sodium intake to help manage blood pressure. Choosing fresh, whole foods and minimizing the use of processed or packaged foods can contribute to reduced sodium consumption.

- **Managing Portion Sizes:** Controlling portion sizes supports weight management and helps regulate blood sugar levels. Seniors can work with dietitians to create personalized meal plans that align with their dietary preferences and health goals.

Regular Physical Activity: Engaging in regular physical activity is beneficial for both diabetes management and cardiovascular health. Seniors should:

- **Choose Enjoyable Activities:** Incorporating enjoyable activities, such as walking, swimming, or gardening, makes it more likely for seniors to adhere to a regular exercise routine.

- **Prioritize Aerobic Exercise:** Aerobic exercises, such as brisk walking, cycling, or swimming, enhance cardiovascular fitness and help control blood sugar levels.

- **Include Strength Training:** Strength training exercises, using resistance bands or weights, can improve muscle strength and contribute to overall physical well-being.

Maintaining a Healthy Weight: Weight management is integral to cardiovascular health for seniors with diabetes. Achieving and maintaining a healthy weight involves:

- **Setting Realistic Goals:** Seniors should work with healthcare providers to set realistic weight loss or maintenance goals based on their health status.

- **Monitoring Portion Sizes:** Being mindful of portion sizes and practicing mindful eating can contribute to weight management.

- **Seeking Support:** Engaging with support networks, such as healthcare professionals, dietitians, or support groups, can provide guidance and encouragement.

Blood Sugar Monitoring and Medication Adherence: Effective diabetes management is a cornerstone of cardiovascular health. Seniors should:

- **Monitor Blood Sugar Levels Regularly:** Regular blood sugar monitoring allows seniors to track their levels and make timely adjustments to their treatment plans.

- **Adhere to Medication Plans:** Taking medications as prescribed by healthcare providers is essential for maintaining optimal blood sugar control and preventing complications.

Regular Health Check-ups: Regular health check-ups provide opportunities for proactive management and early intervention. Seniors should:

- **Schedule Regular Appointments:** Routine visits to healthcare providers allow for the monitoring of blood pressure, blood sugar levels, and overall cardiovascular health.

- **Discuss Concerns and Symptoms:** Seniors should communicate openly with their healthcare providers about any concerns or symptoms related to their heart health.

Stress Management and Mental Well-being: The connection between mental well-being and heart health should not be overlooked. Seniors should:

- **Practice Stress-Reducing Activities:** Engaging in activities such as meditation, deep breathing exercises, or hobbies can help manage stress levels.

- **Seek Support for Mental Health:** Seniors should prioritize mental well-being and seek support if they experience feelings of anxiety or depression.

Avoiding Smoking and Limiting Alcohol Intake: Smoking and excessive alcohol consumption are detrimental to heart health. Seniors should:

- **Quit Smoking:** Smoking is a major risk factor for cardiovascular disease. Quitting smoking has immediate and long-term benefits for heart health.

- **Moderate Alcohol Consumption:** If seniors choose to consume alcohol, they should do so in moderation, following recommended guidelines and avoiding excessive intake.

Implementing these lifestyle strategies requires commitment and ongoing effort, but the benefits extend beyond cardiovascular health. Seniors with diabetes can experience improved overall well-being, enhanced quality of life, and a reduced risk of complications through the adoption of heart-healthy habits.

The intersection of diabetes and cardiovascular health demands a multifaceted approach for seniors. By understanding the impact of diabetes on the heart and embracing lifestyle strategies that prioritize heart health, seniors can navigate their diabetes journey with resilience. Collaboration with healthcare providers, regular monitoring, and proactive lifestyle modifications contribute to the prevention and effective management of cardiovascular complications, ensuring that seniors with diabetes can lead fulfilling and heart-healthy lives.

5.2 Kidney and Eye Health

Seniors with diabetes are at an increased risk of developing complications that affect the kidneys and eyes. This section delves into the intricacies of diabetes-related kidney disease and diabetic retinopathy, providing insights into their impact and offering preventive measures for kidney and eye health in seniors.

5.2.1 Diabetes and Kidney Disease

Diabetes is a leading cause of kidney disease, emphasizing the need for proactive measures to preserve kidney health in seniors with diabetes. Understanding the relationship between diabetes and kidney disease is essential for prevention and management.

Diabetic Nephropathy: Diabetic nephropathy, or diabetes-related kidney disease, is a progressive condition characterized by damage to the kidneys' filtering units (glomeruli). The intricate network of blood vessels in the kidneys becomes impaired, leading to the leakage of essential proteins into the urine. Over time, this can result in decreased kidney function.

Risk Factors for Diabetic Nephropathy: Several factors contribute to the development and progression of diabetic nephropathy in seniors:

1. **Duration of Diabetes:** The longer an individual has diabetes, the higher the risk of developing kidney complications.

2. **Poorly Controlled Blood Sugar Levels:** Inadequate control of blood sugar levels accelerates the progression of diabetic nephropathy.

3. **High Blood Pressure:** Hypertension is a significant risk factor for kidney disease in individuals with diabetes.

4. **Genetic Predisposition:** Some individuals may have a genetic predisposition to kidney disease.

5. **Smoking:** Smoking can exacerbate the impact of diabetes on kidney health.

Preventing Diabetic Nephropathy: Preventive measures play a crucial role in preserving kidney health for seniors with diabetes:

1. **Blood Sugar Control:** Maintaining optimal blood sugar levels through regular monitoring and adherence to treatment plans is fundamental in preventing diabetic nephropathy.

2. **Blood Pressure Management:** Seniors should work with their healthcare providers to control and manage hypertension through lifestyle modifications and medications if necessary.

3. **Regular Kidney Function Monitoring:** Routine tests, such as blood tests to measure creatinine and glomerular filtration rate (GFR), can help monitor kidney function. Early detection allows for timely intervention.

4. **Healthy Lifestyle Habits:** Adopting a healthy lifestyle that includes a balanced diet, regular physical activity,

and avoidance of smoking contributes to overall kidney health.

5. **Medication Adherence:** Taking medications as prescribed, including those for blood sugar and blood pressure control, is vital in preventing kidney complications.

6. **Regular Health Check-ups:** Regular visits to healthcare providers provide opportunities for monitoring kidney function and adjusting treatment plans as needed.

Managing Diabetic Nephropathy: If diabetic nephropathy has already developed, management strategies focus on slowing its progression and preventing further complications:

1. **Blood Pressure Control:** Tight control of blood pressure is crucial to slow the progression of kidney disease. Medications, dietary changes, and lifestyle modifications may be recommended.

2. **Medication Adjustments:** Healthcare providers may adjust medications, including those for diabetes management, to protect kidney function.

3. **Protein Restriction:** In advanced stages of kidney disease, restricting protein intake may be recommended to reduce the workload on the kidneys.

4. **Dialysis or Kidney Transplant:** In severe cases of diabetic nephropathy, when kidney function is significantly impaired, dialysis or kidney transplant may be considered.

Seniors with diabetes should actively engage with their healthcare providers to monitor and manage kidney health effectively. By addressing risk factors and implementing preventive measures, they can significantly reduce the likelihood of diabetic nephropathy and its complications.

5.2.2 Diabetic Retinopathy and Vision Care

Diabetic retinopathy is a diabetes-related complication that affects the eyes, potentially leading to vision impairment or blindness. Understanding the dynamics of diabetic retinopathy and adopting preventive measures is crucial for maintaining optimal vision in seniors with diabetes.

Diabetic Retinopathy: Diabetic retinopathy is a condition that affects the blood vessels in the retina, the light-sensitive tissue at the back of the eye. Elevated blood sugar levels over time can damage the small blood vessels in the retina, leading to various stages of diabetic retinopathy:

1. **Mild Nonproliferative Retinopathy:** Early stage, characterized by small areas of balloon-like swelling in the retina's blood vessels.

2. **Moderate Nonproliferative Retinopathy:** Blood vessels that nourish the retina become blocked.

3. **Severe Nonproliferative Retinopathy:** More blood vessels are blocked, depriving the retina of its blood supply.

4. **Proliferative Retinopathy:** New blood vessels begin to grow on the retina, but they are fragile and can lead to bleeding, retinal detachment, and vision loss.

Risk Factors for Diabetic Retinopathy: Several factors contribute to the development and progression of diabetic retinopathy in seniors:

1. **Duration of Diabetes:** The longer an individual has diabetes, the higher the risk of developing diabetic retinopathy.

2. **Poorly Controlled Blood Sugar Levels:** Inadequate control of blood sugar levels increases the risk and severity of diabetic retinopathy.

3. **Hypertension:** High blood pressure is a significant risk factor for diabetic retinopathy.

4. **Genetic Predisposition:** Individuals with a family history of diabetic retinopathy may be at a higher risk.

5. **Pregnancy:** Pregnant individuals with diabetes may experience an accelerated onset or progression of diabetic retinopathy.

Preventing Diabetic Retinopathy: Preventive measures are crucial in preserving vision and preventing the progression of diabetic retinopathy:

1. **Blood Sugar Control:** Maintaining optimal blood sugar levels is fundamental in preventing and managing diabetic retinopathy. Regular monitoring and adherence to treatment plans are essential.

2. **Blood Pressure Management:** Seniors should work with their healthcare providers to control and manage hypertension to reduce the risk of diabetic retinopathy.

3. **Regular Eye Exams:** Routine eye exams, including dilated eye examinations, allow for the early detection of diabetic retinopathy. Early intervention can prevent or delay vision loss.

4. **Lifestyle Modifications:** Adopting a healthy lifestyle that includes a balanced diet, regular physical activity, and avoidance of smoking contributes to overall eye health.

5. **Medication Adherence:** Taking medications as prescribed, including those for blood sugar and blood pressure control, is vital in preventing diabetic retinopathy.

6. **Protecting Eyes from Sunlight:** Wearing sunglasses that block ultraviolet (UV) rays helps protect the eyes from potential damage.

Managing Diabetic Retinopathy: If diabetic retinopathy has already developed, management strategies focus on slowing its progression and preventing further vision loss:

1. **Laser Therapy:** Laser therapy may be used to seal or shrink abnormal blood vessels in the retina, preventing further bleeding and fluid leakage.

2. **Intravitreal Injections:** Medications may be injected into the vitreous gel of the eye to slow the growth of abnormal blood vessels and reduce swelling.

3. **Vitrectomy:** In advanced cases where there is significant bleeding into the vitreous gel, a vitrectomy may be performed to remove blood and scar tissue.

4. **Regular Eye Monitoring:** Seniors with diabetic retinopathy should have regular eye check-ups to monitor the progression of the condition and adjust treatment plans accordingly.

Seniors with diabetes should prioritize their eye health by proactively engaging with healthcare providers, attending regular eye exams, and adopting preventive measures. Through these efforts, the onset and progression of diabetic retinopathy can be effectively managed, preserving vision and overall quality of life.

Kidney and eye health are integral components of comprehensive diabetes care for seniors. By understanding the specific risks and adopting preventive measures, seniors can actively engage in preserving the health of these vital organs. Collaborative efforts with healthcare providers, regular monitoring, and adherence to lifestyle modifications contribute to effective prevention and management of complications, ensuring that seniors with diabetes can lead fulfilling and healthy lives.

5.3 Neuropathy and Foot Care

Neuropathy, or nerve damage, is a prevalent complication of diabetes that can have a profound impact on a senior's quality of life. Additionally, foot-related problems can escalate, posing significant risks. This section delves into the prevention and management of neuropathic complications and underscores the vital importance of proper foot care for seniors with diabetes.

5.3.1 Preventing and Managing Neuropathic Complications

Neuropathy, characterized by nerve damage, is a common complication of diabetes, affecting various nerves throughout the body. Seniors with diabetes need to be proactive in preventing and managing neuropathic complications to maintain optimal function and well-being.

Types of Diabetic Neuropathy:

1. **Peripheral Neuropathy:** This is the most common form of diabetic neuropathy, affecting the nerves of the feet and legs first, and then progressing to the hands and arms. Symptoms may include numbness, tingling, burning sensations, and pain.

2. **Autonomic Neuropathy:** This type affects the nerves that control involuntary bodily functions, leading to issues with digestion, heart rate, blood pressure, and bladder function.

3. **Proximal Neuropathy:** This type is characterized by pain in the thighs, hips, or buttocks and can lead to weakness in the legs.

4. **Focal Neuropathy:** This type results in sudden weakness or pain in specific nerves or groups of nerves, often in the head, torso, or leg.

Preventing Neuropathic Complications:

Preventive measures play a crucial role in minimizing the impact of neuropathy on seniors with diabetes. Key strategies include:

1. **Blood Sugar Control:** Maintaining stable blood sugar levels is fundamental in preventing and slowing the progression of neuropathy. Seniors should adhere to their treatment plans, monitor blood sugar regularly, and make necessary adjustments.

2. **Regular Exercise:** Physical activity promotes circulation and nerve health. Seniors should engage in exercises that are safe and suitable for their fitness levels, such as walking, swimming, or gentle stretches.

3. **Balanced Diet:** A diet rich in nutrients, especially B vitamins, is beneficial for nerve health. Seniors should work with dietitians to ensure they are receiving adequate nutrition.

4. **Quit Smoking:** Smoking narrows blood vessels and can exacerbate nerve damage. Quitting smoking has immediate and long-term benefits for nerve health.

5. **Limit Alcohol Intake:** Excessive alcohol consumption can contribute to nerve damage. Seniors should follow recommended guidelines for alcohol consumption.

6. **Regular Health Check-ups:** Regular monitoring by healthcare providers allows for the early detection of neuropathic symptoms. Adjustments to treatment plans can be made promptly.

Managing Neuropathic Complications:

If neuropathic complications have already developed, effective management is crucial to alleviate symptoms and prevent further deterioration. Management strategies include:

1. **Medications:** Various medications, such as pain relievers, anticonvulsants, and antidepressants, may be prescribed to manage symptoms.

2. **Physical Therapy:** Physical therapy can help improve strength, flexibility, and balance, contributing to better overall function and reducing the risk of falls.

3. **Foot Care:** Proper foot care is essential in managing neuropathy, as foot-related issues are common in individuals with diabetes. Regular monitoring, appropriate footwear, and preventive measures can prevent complications.

4. **Pain Management Techniques:** Non-pharmacological approaches, such as massage, acupuncture, or relaxation techniques, may help manage neuropathic pain.

5. **Blood Pressure Control:** Managing blood pressure is crucial, as hypertension can exacerbate neuropathic complications. Seniors should work closely with healthcare providers to control blood pressure.

By incorporating these preventive and management strategies into their daily lives, seniors can mitigate the impact of neuropathy, promoting better overall well-being and preserving functional abilities.

5.3.2 Importance of Foot Care

Foot care is of paramount importance for seniors with diabetes, as complications related to the feet can have severe consequences. Proper foot care not only prevents issues but also contributes to the overall management of diabetes and the preservation of mobility.

Common Foot Issues in Diabetes:

1. **Peripheral Neuropathy:** Nerve damage can lead to loss of sensation in the feet, making it difficult to detect injuries or irritations.

2. **Peripheral Artery Disease (PAD):** Reduced blood flow to the feet increases the risk of infections and delays the healing of wounds.

3. **Foot Ulcers:** Poorly managed diabetes can lead to the development of foot ulcers, which are open sores that can become infected and challenging to heal.

4. **Calluses and Corns:** Pressure points on the feet can result in the formation of calluses and corns, which, if not managed, can lead to complications.

5. **Ingrown Toenails:** Improper trimming or tight footwear can cause toenails to grow into the surrounding skin, leading to infection.

Preventive Foot Care Measures:

Seniors with diabetes can take proactive steps to prevent foot-related complications:

1. **Daily Foot Inspections:** Regularly inspecting the feet for cuts, sores, blisters, or any abnormalities is crucial. Seniors should use a mirror or seek assistance if visibility is challenging.

2. **Proper Footwear:** Wearing comfortable, well-fitting shoes is essential. Specialized diabetic shoes may be recommended for those with foot issues.

3. **Moisturizing and Nail Care:** Keeping the feet moisturized helps prevent dry skin and cracking. Nail care involves trimming toenails straight across to prevent ingrown nails.

4. **Avoiding Barefoot Walking:** Seniors should avoid walking barefoot to minimize the risk of injuries.

5. **Regular Foot Exams:** Healthcare providers should conduct regular foot exams to identify potential issues and provide appropriate interventions.

6. **Blood Sugar Control:** Stable blood sugar levels contribute to better overall foot health. Seniors should monitor blood sugar regularly and adhere to treatment plans.

7. **Smoking Cessation:** Quitting smoking is beneficial for vascular health, reducing the risk of peripheral artery disease.

8. **Managing Peripheral Artery Disease:** Seniors with PAD may need additional measures to improve blood flow to the feet, such as medications or lifestyle changes.

Prompt Intervention for Foot Issues:

If seniors notice any foot-related issues, prompt intervention is crucial:

1. **Avoid Self-Treatment:** Seniors should refrain from attempting to self-treat foot problems, especially if there are cuts, sores, or signs of infection.

2. **Seek Medical Attention:** Any signs of infection, non-healing wounds, or changes in foot sensation should

prompt immediate medical attention. Healthcare providers can address issues before they escalate.

3. **Foot Care Education:** Seniors should receive education on proper foot care from healthcare providers, including guidance on daily practices and recognizing potential problems.

4. **Coordination with Podiatrists:** Regular visits to podiatrists, who specialize in foot care, can be beneficial for seniors with diabetes. Podiatrists can provide specialized care and advice tailored to individual needs.

The Role of Regular Physical Activity:

In addition to foot-specific measures, regular physical activity contributes to overall health and can have positive effects on foot circulation. Seniors should engage in activities that are safe and suitable for their fitness level, taking into consideration any existing foot issues.

By prioritizing foot care and incorporating preventive measures into their daily routines, seniors with diabetes can significantly reduce the risk of foot-related complications. Proper foot care is an integral component of diabetes management, promoting mobility, independence, and overall well-being.

Neuropathy and foot care are essential aspects of comprehensive diabetes care for seniors. By understanding the intricacies of neuropathic complications, adopting preventive measures, and prioritizing foot health, seniors can navigate their diabetes journey with resilience. Collaborative efforts with healthcare providers, regular monitoring, and proactive lifestyle modifications contribute to the prevention and effective management of complications, ensuring that seniors with diabetes can lead fulfilling and healthy lives.

Chapter 6:

Building a Support System

Living with diabetes as a senior comes with its unique challenges, and having a robust support system is crucial for overall well-being. This chapter explores the significance of emotional support and provides insights into leveraging relationships with family and friends, as well as the benefits of participating in support groups and seeking counseling.

6.1 Importance of Emotional Support

Emotional support is a cornerstone of effective diabetes management, especially for seniors navigating the complexities of the condition. Understanding the importance of emotional well-being and having a strong support system can significantly impact a senior's ability to cope with the challenges of diabetes.

6.1.1 Family and Friends

Family and friends play a pivotal role in providing emotional support to seniors with diabetes. The impact of a positive and understanding social network goes beyond emotional well-being, influencing lifestyle choices, treatment adherence, and overall quality of life.

Understanding the Role of Family and Friends:

1. **Emotional Understanding:** Living with diabetes can be emotionally taxing. Family and friends who understand the emotional toll of the condition can provide a safe space for seniors to express their feelings, concerns, and frustrations.

2. **Encouragement and Motivation:** Positive reinforcement and words of encouragement can motivate seniors to adhere to their treatment plans, make healthy lifestyle choices, and stay resilient in the face of challenges.

3. **Practical Support:** Practical assistance, such as helping with meal preparation, transportation to medical appointments, or participating in physical activities, eases the daily burden and fosters a sense of togetherness.

4. **Reducing Isolation:** Diabetes management can sometimes lead to feelings of isolation. Regular interaction with family and friends helps combat loneliness and creates a supportive environment.

Building Effective Communication:

1. **Open Dialogue:** Open communication is essential. Seniors should feel comfortable discussing their diabetes-related concerns, and family and friends should actively listen and provide constructive feedback.

2. **Educating Loved Ones:** Providing education about diabetes to family and friends helps them understand the condition better. This knowledge enables them to offer more meaningful support and participate actively in the senior's care.

3. **Setting Realistic Expectations:** Setting realistic expectations is crucial. Both seniors and their loved ones should acknowledge that living with diabetes requires adjustments and that challenges may arise.

Understanding and accepting these challenges collectively can strengthen the support system.

Celebrating Achievements Together:

1. **Recognizing Milestones:** Celebrating achievements, no matter how small, is essential. Whether it's reaching a blood sugar target, adopting a healthier lifestyle, or successfully managing a specific aspect of diabetes, acknowledging these milestones reinforces positive behavior.

2. **Participating in Shared Activities:** Engaging in shared activities fosters a sense of normalcy and joy. Whether it's participating in family gatherings, outings, or hobbies, these experiences contribute to emotional well-being and strengthen familial bonds.

3. **Inclusive Health Initiatives:** Encouraging overall health initiatives benefits everyone. Families can embark on healthy eating plans, participate in regular exercise routines together, and collectively adopt a wellness-focused lifestyle.

6.1.2 Support Groups and Counseling

Beyond familial and friendship networks, seniors with diabetes can benefit significantly from engaging with support groups and seeking counseling. These avenues offer specialized assistance, provide a sense of community, and address specific emotional needs related to diabetes management.

The Role of Support Groups:

1. **Shared Experiences:** Support groups bring together individuals who share similar experiences. Seniors can

relate to others facing the daily challenges of diabetes, creating a supportive community.

2. **Information Exchange:** Support groups are valuable platforms for sharing information. Participants can exchange insights, strategies, and practical tips for managing diabetes, enhancing everyone's knowledge base.

3. **Emotional Connection:** The emotional connection fostered in support groups is unique. Seniors can express their feelings without fear of judgment, receiving empathy and understanding from those who truly comprehend the nuances of living with diabetes.

4. **Motivation and Inspiration:** Seeing others successfully manage diabetes can be motivating and inspiring. Support group members can serve as role models, offering hope and encouragement to seniors who may be facing difficulties.

Benefits of Professional Counseling:

1. **Emotional Well-being:** Professional counseling provides a confidential space for seniors to explore their emotions, fears, and challenges related to diabetes. A trained counselor can offer guidance on coping strategies and emotional well-being.

2. **Stress Management:** Living with diabetes can be stressful, and counseling equips seniors with effective stress management techniques. Learning how to navigate stress positively is crucial for overall health.

3. **Coping with Change:** Diabetes often requires lifestyle adjustments. Counseling helps seniors navigate these

changes, providing tools to adapt to new routines, dietary requirements, and treatment plans.

4. **Family Dynamics:** Counselors can facilitate family discussions, addressing the dynamics of living with diabetes. This can enhance communication, understanding, and collaboration within the family unit.

Finding the Right Support System:

1. **Researching Local Support Groups:** Seniors can explore local community centers, healthcare facilities, or online platforms to find diabetes-specific support groups. These groups may focus on particular aspects of diabetes, such as type 2 diabetes or diabetes in seniors.

2. **Seeking Referrals from Healthcare Providers:** Healthcare providers often have insights into local support groups and can provide recommendations based on a senior's specific needs and preferences.

3. **Online Resources:** Virtual support groups and counseling services are accessible through online platforms. These resources offer flexibility and convenience, allowing seniors to connect with others and access professional guidance from the comfort of their homes.

4. **Checking with Diabetes Organizations:** Diabetes organizations often organize or endorse support groups. Seniors can explore options provided by reputable diabetes organizations, ensuring a reliable and informed network.

Overcoming Stigma Associated with Counseling:

1. **Normalizing Mental Health Discussions:** Encouraging open discussions about mental health reduces the stigma associated with seeking counseling. Seniors should recognize that mental and emotional well-being is an integral part of overall health.

2. **Highlighting Positive Outcomes:** Sharing success stories of individuals who have benefited from counseling can inspire others to seek professional support. Understanding that counseling can lead to positive outcomes reinforces its importance.

3. **Emphasizing Personal Growth:** Counseling is not solely about addressing challenges; it also fosters personal growth. Seniors can view counseling as an opportunity for self-discovery, skill development, and resilience-building.

4. **Family Involvement:** Involving family members in the counseling process can destigmatize seeking professional help. Family support is crucial, and their active participation can contribute to the overall success of counseling.

Continued Engagement:

1. **Consistent Participation:** Seniors should commit to consistent participation in support groups or counseling sessions. Regular engagement fosters a sense of belonging and maximizes the benefits of emotional support.

2. **Adapting to Changing Needs:** As needs evolve, seniors may find that their preferences for support

groups or counseling change. Being adaptable and exploring different avenues ensures a tailored and effective support system.

3. **Feedback and Communication:** Providing feedback to support group facilitators or counselors helps tailor the experience to individual needs. Seniors should feel empowered to communicate their preferences and expectations.

4. **Combining Support Systems:** Seniors can leverage both familial support and professional resources concurrently. The combination of family and friend networks with the insights gained from support groups and counseling creates a comprehensive support system.

Building a robust support system is an integral aspect of effectively managing diabetes as a senior. The emotional support provided by family and friends, coupled with the unique benefits of support groups and counseling, contributes to a holistic approach to diabetes management. Seniors are encouraged to actively seek and cultivate these support systems, recognizing the positive impact they can have on emotional well-being, treatment adherence, and overall quality of life. Collaborative efforts between seniors, their loved ones, and healthcare providers create a resilient foundation for navigating the challenges of diabetes in their senior years.

6.2 Communicating with Healthcare Professionals

Effectively communicating with healthcare professionals is a cornerstone of successful diabetes management. Seniors with diabetes should actively engage with their healthcare team, fostering open communication, building relationships, and advocating for their specific health needs. This section delves into the intricacies of this vital aspect of diabetes care.

6.2.1 Building a Relationship with Your Healthcare Team

Establishing a strong relationship with the healthcare team is foundational to effective diabetes management. The healthcare team comprises various professionals, including primary care physicians, endocrinologists, nurses, dietitians, and pharmacists. Building a collaborative and trusting relationship with each member enhances the quality of care and contributes to better health outcomes.

Elements of a Strong Relationship:

1. **Open Communication:** Seniors should feel comfortable expressing their concerns, asking questions, and providing feedback. Healthcare professionals, in turn, should actively listen, offer clear explanations, and address any uncertainties.

2. **Mutual Trust:** Trust is a two-way street. Seniors should trust the expertise of their healthcare professionals, and healthcare professionals should trust the seniors' ability to actively participate in their care.

3. **Shared Decision-Making:** Informed decision-making involves collaboration between seniors and healthcare professionals. Both parties should actively participate in discussions about treatment plans, lifestyle modifications, and goal-setting.

4. **Consistency in Care:** A consistent approach to care ensures that seniors receive comprehensive and cohesive support. Consistency includes regular check-ups, follow-ups, and timely adjustments to treatment plans as needed.

Effective Communication Strategies:

1. **Prepare for Appointments:** Seniors should prepare for appointments by noting down questions, concerns, and observations. This ensures that all relevant topics are covered during the limited time of the appointment.

2. **Be Honest and Transparent:** Openness about symptoms, lifestyle habits, and any challenges faced is crucial. Honest communication provides healthcare professionals with valuable insights for personalized care.

3. **Understand Medical Jargon:** Healthcare professionals should communicate in a language that seniors can understand. Clear explanations, avoidance of excessive medical jargon, and the use of visual aids contribute to effective communication.

4. **Utilize Technology:** Technology can enhance communication. Seniors can use communication apps, patient portals, or wearable devices to share relevant health data with their healthcare team, facilitating remote monitoring and timely interventions.

The Role of Different Healthcare Professionals:

1. **Primary Care Physicians:** Primary care physicians play a central role in diabetes management. They oversee

overall health, conduct regular check-ups, and coordinate with specialists when needed.

2. **Endocrinologists:** Endocrinologists specialize in hormonal disorders, including diabetes. Seniors may consult endocrinologists for specialized guidance on diabetes management.

3. **Nurses:** Nurses provide essential support in diabetes care, including administering medications, conducting health assessments, and offering educational resources.

4. **Dietitians:** Dietitians play a crucial role in developing personalized meal plans, offering nutritional guidance, and addressing dietary concerns specific to diabetes management.

5. **Pharmacists:** Pharmacists contribute by ensuring medication adherence, providing information on potential drug interactions, and offering guidance on proper medication administration.

Building Trust Over Time:

1. **Consistent Communication:** Regular and consistent communication fosters trust. Seniors should attend scheduled appointments, follow up on recommendations, and promptly communicate any changes in their health status.

2. **Feedback Loop:** An ongoing feedback loop ensures that both seniors and healthcare professionals are actively engaged in the care process. Seniors should provide feedback on their experiences and share any concerns or challenges faced.

3. **Shared Goal Setting:** Collaboratively setting health goals promotes a sense of shared responsibility. Seniors and healthcare professionals should align on achievable objectives and milestones.

4. **Adaptability:** Healthcare is dynamic, and adjustments to treatment plans may be necessary. Seniors should feel confident in their healthcare team's adaptability and responsiveness to evolving health needs.

6.2.2 Advocating for Your Health Needs

Advocacy is an empowering aspect of diabetes management for seniors. Advocating for one's health needs involves actively participating in decision-making, expressing preferences, and ensuring that individual concerns are addressed. Seniors should view themselves as equal partners in their care, capable of contributing valuable insights to the healthcare decision-making process.

Elements of Effective Health Advocacy:

1. **Self-Knowledge:** Understanding one's health condition, treatment plan, and personal preferences is foundational. Seniors should actively educate themselves about diabetes and be aware of their individual health goals.

2. **Clear Communication:** Advocacy begins with clear and assertive communication. Seniors should express their needs, concerns, and preferences openly, ensuring that healthcare professionals have a comprehensive understanding of their health context.

3. **Informed Decision-Making:** Seniors should actively participate in decision-making processes. This includes

discussing treatment options, and potential side effects, and actively contributing to the development of personalized care plans.

4. **Questioning and Clarification:** Seniors should feel empowered to ask questions and seek clarification. Understanding the rationale behind treatment decisions and seeking additional information contributes to informed decision-making.

Navigating Healthcare Systems:

1. **Understanding Insurance Coverage:** Seniors should have a clear understanding of their insurance coverage, including the specifics of diabetes-related services and medications. This knowledge aids in making informed healthcare choices.

2. **Accessing Community Resources:** Community resources, such as local health clinics, diabetes education programs, and support groups, can complement healthcare services. Seniors should explore available resources to enhance their support network.

3. **Seeking Second Opinions:** In complex healthcare situations, seeking a second opinion can provide additional perspectives and insights. Seniors should feel comfortable consulting other healthcare professionals for input on their care.

4. **Utilizing Patient Advocacy Services:** Patient advocacy services can assist seniors in navigating complex healthcare systems, addressing insurance issues, and ensuring that their rights are upheld. These

services offer support in understanding and navigating the healthcare landscape.

Overcoming Barriers to Advocacy:

1. **Overcoming Age-Related Stereotypes:** Seniors may encounter age-related stereotypes that assume a passive role in healthcare decision-making. Actively challenging and overcoming these stereotypes is crucial for effective advocacy.

2. **Empowering Caregivers:** Seniors can involve caregivers in the advocacy process, ensuring that there is a support system in place. Caregivers can provide additional insights and assistance in navigating healthcare systems.

3. **Cultural Sensitivity:** Cultural factors may influence healthcare dynamics. Seniors should advocate for culturally sensitive care, ensuring that their values, preferences, and cultural considerations are respected.

4. **Addressing Communication Barriers:** Language barriers or hearing impairments can pose challenges to effective communication. Seniors should advocate for accessible communication methods, such as interpreters or written materials, to ensure understanding.

Collaborative Decision-Making:

1. **Involving Family Members:** In cases where family members are actively involved in a senior's care, their perspectives and insights should be considered. Collaborative decision-making involves incorporating the preferences of both seniors and their families.

2. **Shared Goal Setting:** Establishing shared health goals ensures that advocacy efforts align with overall health objectives. Seniors and healthcare professionals should jointly set realistic and achievable goals.

3. **Advocacy in Emergency Situations:** Seniors should communicate their specific health needs to emergency responders, ensuring that they receive appropriate care in emergencies. Wearing a medical alert bracelet with relevant information can be beneficial.

4. **Documentation and Communication:** Keeping a health journal or documentation of symptoms, concerns, and questions can aid in effective communication during healthcare appointments. Seniors can share this information with their healthcare team to facilitate comprehensive care.

Effective communication with healthcare professionals and advocating for one's health needs are integral components of successful diabetes management for seniors. Building strong relationships with the healthcare team, actively participating in care decisions, and navigating healthcare systems through advocacy contribute to a personalized and empowering approach to diabetes care. Seniors are encouraged to embrace their role as active partners in their health journey, recognizing the value of their insights and the positive impact of collaborative efforts with healthcare professionals. By fostering open communication and advocating for individual health needs, seniors can navigate the complexities of diabetes with resilience and confidence.

Chapter 7:

Emotional Well-being and Coping Strategies for Seniors with Diabetes

Diabetes not only affects the physical well-being of seniors but also takes a toll on their emotional health. This chapter delves into the emotional challenges faced by seniors with diabetes and provides valuable insights into coping strategies. It emphasizes the importance of addressing mental health concerns, managing stress and anxiety related to diabetes, and building a supportive network for enhanced emotional well-being.

7.1 Addressing Emotional Challenges and Mental Health

Emotional challenges are an inherent aspect of living with diabetes, particularly for seniors who may be navigating additional life changes and health considerations. Addressing these emotional challenges and prioritizing mental health is crucial for comprehensive diabetes care.

Understanding the Emotional Impact of Diabetes:

1. Fear and Anxiety: The chronic nature of diabetes can evoke fear and anxiety. Seniors may worry about the progression of the condition, potential complications, and the impact on their overall quality of life.

2. Depression: Living with a chronic illness like diabetes can contribute to feelings of sadness and depression. Coping with daily management, lifestyle changes, and potential limitations can be emotionally taxing.

3. Grief and Loss: Seniors may experience a sense of loss, especially if diabetes necessitates lifestyle changes or restricts activities they once enjoyed. Grieving the perceived loss of normalcy is a valid emotional response.

4. Stigma and Isolation: Stigmatization associated with diabetes can lead to feelings of isolation. Seniors may hesitate to share their diagnosis due to fear of judgment or misunderstanding, contributing to a sense of social isolation.

Promoting Mental Health in Seniors:

1. Open Communication: Encouraging open communication about emotional challenges is essential. Seniors should feel comfortable discussing their feelings with healthcare professionals, family members, or friends.

2. Seeking Professional Support: Mental health professionals, such as psychologists or counselors, can provide valuable support. Seniors can benefit from therapy sessions to explore and address the emotional impact of diabetes.

3. Participating in Support Groups: Joining diabetes-specific support groups connects seniors with individuals facing similar emotional challenges. Sharing experiences, gaining insights, and receiving empathy contribute to a sense of belonging.

4. Educating Family and Friends: Family and friends can play a crucial role in supporting a senior's mental

health. Educating them about the emotional impact of diabetes fosters understanding and empathy.

5. Incorporating Relaxation Techniques: Techniques such as deep breathing, meditation, or mindfulness can alleviate stress and promote emotional well-being. Seniors can explore these practices as part of their daily routine.

7.2 Coping with Diabetes-related Stress and Anxiety

Stress and anxiety are common responses to the demands of managing diabetes. Recognizing these challenges and implementing effective coping strategies is essential for seniors to navigate the emotional aspects of their diabetes journey.

Understanding Diabetes-related Stress:

1. Treatment Burden: The daily management of diabetes, including medication adherence, blood sugar monitoring, and dietary restrictions, can contribute to treatment-related stress.

2. Uncertainty and Future Concerns: The uncertainty surrounding the progression of diabetes and the potential for complications can create anxiety about the future. Seniors may worry about their health and independence.

3. Social and Lifestyle Adjustments: Diabetes often requires lifestyle adjustments, such as changes in diet and physical activity. Seniors may find these adjustments challenging, leading to stress and feelings of restriction.

Effective Coping Strategies:

1. Time Management and Routine: Establishing a consistent routine for diabetes management can reduce stress. Seniors should allocate specific times for medication, meals, and other diabetes-related activities.

2. Goal Setting: Setting achievable and realistic goals provides a sense of accomplishment. Seniors can focus on specific aspects of diabetes management and celebrate milestones along the way.

3. Problem-solving Skills: Developing effective problem-solving skills enhances a senior's ability to navigate challenges. Identifying potential stressors and implementing proactive solutions contributes to a sense of control.

4. Regular Physical Activity: Exercise is a powerful stress reliever. Seniors should engage in regular physical activity, incorporating exercises that align with their fitness levels and preferences.

5. Social Engagement: Maintaining social connections is crucial. Seniors should actively engage with family, friends, and support groups, fostering a sense of community and reducing feelings of isolation.

7.3 Building a Supportive Network and Engaging in Self-Care

Building a supportive network and prioritizing self-care are essential components of fostering emotional well-being for seniors with diabetes. Creating a robust support system and incorporating self-care practices contribute to resilience in the face of diabetes-related challenges.

The Importance of a Supportive Network:

1. Family and Friends: The support of family and friends is invaluable. Seniors should communicate their needs and involve loved ones in their diabetes journey, fostering a collaborative and understanding environment.

2. Support Groups: Diabetes-specific support groups connect seniors with individuals who share similar experiences. These groups provide a platform for sharing insights, gaining advice, and receiving emotional support.

3. Healthcare Team: The healthcare team plays a central role in the support network. Seniors should actively engage with healthcare professionals, seeking guidance on emotional well-being and addressing mental health concerns.

Engaging in Self-Care Practices:

1. Prioritizing Rest and Sleep: Adequate rest and quality sleep are essential for emotional well-being. Seniors should prioritize a consistent sleep routine and create a conducive sleep environment.

2. Healthy Nutrition: Proper nutrition not only supports physical health but also influences mood and energy levels. Seniors should focus on a balanced diet that aligns with their diabetes management plan.

3. Creative Outlets: Engaging in creative activities, such as art, writing, or music, provides a positive outlet for emotions. Seniors can explore hobbies that bring joy and fulfillment.

4. Mindfulness and Relaxation: Practicing mindfulness and relaxation techniques contributes to emotional resilience. Seniors can incorporate practices like meditation or gentle yoga into their daily routines.

5. Setting Boundaries: Establishing boundaries in personal and social interactions is crucial. Seniors should communicate their needs and prioritize activities that align with their well-being.

Cultivating Resilience:

1. Accepting Imperfections: Perfectionism can contribute to stress. Seniors should embrace the idea that managing diabetes is a continuous journey, allowing room for imperfections and adjustments.

2. Celebrating Achievements: Acknowledging and celebrating achievements, no matter how small, reinforces positive behavior. Seniors should recognize their efforts in diabetes management and overall well-being.

3. Adapting to Change: Flexibility and adaptability are key components of resilience. Seniors should approach changes in health, treatment plans, and lifestyle with a mindset of adaptability.

4. Learning from Challenges: Every challenge presents an opportunity for learning and growth. Seniors can view difficulties as lessons, gaining insights that contribute to their resilience in managing diabetes.

Seeking Professional Guidance:

1. Therapeutic Interventions: In some cases, therapeutic interventions may be beneficial. Seniors can explore counseling or therapy to address specific emotional challenges and develop coping strategies.

2. Collaboration with the Healthcare Team: Open communication with the healthcare team includes discussing emotional well-being. Healthcare professionals can guide resources and interventions to support mental health.

3. Medication Management: In situations where emotional challenges significantly impact daily functioning, medication management may be considered. Seniors should consult with healthcare professionals to explore appropriate options.

Embracing a Holistic Approach:

1. Integration of Mind and Body: Recognizing the interconnectedness of mental and physical health is essential. Seniors should adopt a holistic approach that considers both aspects of their diabetes management journey.

2. Individualized Strategies: Emotional well-being is highly individualized. Seniors should explore and implement strategies that resonate with their preferences, values, and unique needs.

3. Regular Reflection: Periodic self-reflection allows seniors to assess their emotional well-being and make adjustments as needed. Regular check-ins with themselves contribute to ongoing self-awareness.

Addressing the emotional challenges associated with diabetes and implementing effective coping strategies are integral aspects of holistic diabetes care for seniors. By prioritizing mental health, managing stress and anxiety, and building a supportive network, seniors can navigate the emotional nuances of their diabetes journey with resilience and positivity. Embracing self-care practices, cultivating a strong support system, and seeking professional guidance when needed contribute to a comprehensive and empowering approach to emotional well-being. Seniors are encouraged to actively engage in strategies that resonate with them, recognizing the importance of emotional health in fostering a fulfilling and balanced life despite the challenges of living with diabetes.

Chapter 8:

Navigating Senior Living and Diabetes Management

As seniors transition into different living arrangements, managing diabetes becomes a nuanced challenge. This chapter explores the intricacies of diabetes management in assisted living facilities and nursing homes, strategies for maintaining diabetes care while traveling, and financial considerations with valuable resources tailored to senior diabetes care.

8.1 Diabetes Management in Assisted Living Facilities and Nursing Homes

Entering assisted living facilities or nursing homes marks a significant shift in a senior's lifestyle. Effectively managing diabetes in these environments requires collaboration between residents, healthcare professionals, and facility staff. This section addresses the unique considerations and strategies for diabetes care in senior living settings.

Understanding Assisted Living and Nursing Homes:

1. **Diverse Care Models:** Assisted living facilities and nursing homes offer various care models, ranging from minimal assistance to comprehensive medical care. Understanding the specific model and services provided is essential for diabetes management.

2. **Staff Training and Competency:** Assessing the training and competency of facility staff in diabetes care is crucial. Seniors should ensure that staff members are

knowledgeable about diabetes, its management, and potential complications.

3. **Individualized Care Plans:** Developing individualized care plans is fundamental. Seniors should actively participate in creating care plans that align with their diabetes management needs, including medication schedules, dietary preferences, and exercise routines.

Collaboration with Healthcare Professionals:

1. **Communication with the Healthcare Team:** Ongoing communication with the healthcare team is vital. Seniors should coordinate with their primary care physicians, endocrinologists, and other specialists to ensure that their diabetes management plans align with the care provided in the facility.

2. **Regular Health Assessments:** Regular health assessments, including blood sugar monitoring, should be incorporated into the facility's care routine. Seniors should advocate for the inclusion of diabetes-specific assessments in their overall health monitoring.

3. **Medication Management:** Ensuring proper medication management is essential. Seniors should work closely with healthcare professionals and facility staff to maintain medication adherence and monitor for any medication-related issues.

Daily Diabetes Management Strategies:

1. **Meal Planning and Dietary Considerations:** Collaborating with facility nutritionists or dietitians is crucial for meal planning. Seniors should communicate

dietary preferences, restrictions, and any specific considerations related to diabetes-friendly nutrition.

2. **Physical Activity and Exercise Programs:** Participating in facility-sponsored exercise programs or incorporating physical activity into daily routines contributes to diabetes management. Seniors should communicate their fitness levels and preferences to ensure personalized exercise plans.

3. **Monitoring Blood Sugar Levels:** Regular monitoring of blood sugar levels is a cornerstone of diabetes care. Seniors should work with facility staff to establish a schedule for blood sugar checks, ensuring that these checks align with their healthcare recommendations.

4. **Emergency Preparedness:** Establishing emergency protocols specific to diabetes is essential. Seniors should communicate their emergency needs, including access to medications, glucose monitoring devices, and a clear plan for addressing hypoglycemic or hyperglycemic events.

8.2 Traveling and Maintaining Diabetes Care on the Go

Seniors with diabetes often find themselves navigating the challenges of maintaining diabetes care while traveling. Whether it's for leisure, family visits, or other reasons, planning and preparation are key elements to ensure continuity in diabetes management.

Preparation and Planning:

1. **Medication and Supplies Checklist:** Creating a comprehensive checklist for medications and supplies is essential. Seniors should ensure they have an

adequate supply of medications, testing strips, glucose monitoring devices, and any other essential diabetes-related items.

2. **Communication with the Healthcare Team:** Informing the healthcare team about travel plans is crucial. Seniors should consult with their primary care physicians or endocrinologists to discuss potential adjustments to medication schedules, time zone changes, and other considerations.

3. **Insurance Coverage Verification:** Verifying insurance coverage for medications and healthcare services during travel is important. Seniors should contact their insurance providers to understand coverage outside their usual geographical area.

Managing Diabetes While Traveling:

1. **Time Zone Adjustments:** Seniors traveling across time zones should discuss potential adjustments to medication schedules with their healthcare team. Proper planning ensures that insulin or other medications are administered at the appropriate times.

2. **Access to Healthy Food Options:** Identifying and planning for access to healthy food options is essential. Seniors should research dining options at their travel destination and plan meals that align with their dietary requirements.

3. **Hydration and Physical Activity:** Staying hydrated and incorporating physical activity into travel plans is important for overall well-being. Seniors should

prioritize regular water intake and plan for activities that promote circulation and mobility.

4. **Emergency Preparedness:** Having an emergency kit that includes diabetes-specific items is crucial. Seniors should carry a supply of medications, snacks for hypoglycemic events, and information detailing their diabetes management plan in case of emergencies.

8.3 Financial Considerations and Resources for Senior Diabetes Care

The financial aspect of diabetes care is a significant consideration for seniors, impacting access to medications, healthcare services, and supportive resources. This section explores financial considerations and available resources tailored to support seniors in managing the costs associated with diabetes care.

Understanding Financial Considerations:

1. **Medication Costs:** Seniors should be aware of the costs associated with diabetes medications. Exploring generic options, prescription assistance programs and pharmacy discount programs can help mitigate medication expenses.

2. **Health Insurance Coverage:** Understanding health insurance coverage is crucial. Seniors should review their insurance plans to assess coverage for diabetes-related services, medications, and supplies, ensuring that they are aware of any co-pays or out-of-pocket expenses.

3. **Medicare and Medicaid Benefits:** Seniors eligible for Medicare or Medicaid should explore the benefits

available for diabetes care. Understanding coverage options, preventive services, and eligibility criteria can guide seniors in maximizing their benefits.

Accessing Supportive Resources:

1. **Patient Assistance Programs:** Many pharmaceutical companies offer patient assistance programs to support individuals with limited financial means. Seniors can explore these programs to access discounted or free medications.

2. **Community Health Clinics:** Community health clinics may provide affordable healthcare services, including diabetes screenings, education, and management. Seniors can inquire about sliding fee scales and available resources.

3. **Nonprofit Organizations:** Numerous nonprofit organizations focus on supporting individuals with diabetes. These organizations may offer financial assistance, educational resources, and community programs tailored to seniors.

4. **Local Health Departments:** Local health departments often provide resources for diabetes management. Seniors can inquire about educational workshops, support groups, and available services in their community.

Financial Planning for Diabetes Care:

1. **Budgeting for Medications and Supplies:** Seniors should incorporate medication and supply costs into their overall budget. Planning for these expenses

ensures that financial resources are allocated appropriately for diabetes care.

2. **Exploring Generic Alternatives:** In consultation with healthcare professionals, seniors can explore generic alternatives for medications. Generic options may offer cost savings while maintaining the effectiveness of treatment.

3. **Utilizing Preventive Services:** Medicare and other insurance plans often cover preventive services related to diabetes care. Seniors should schedule regular screenings, check-ups, and preventive care appointments to address potential issues early.

4. **Seeking Financial Counseling:** Financial counseling services can assist seniors in navigating the complexities of healthcare costs. Seniors can explore available resources for financial counseling to gain insights into budgeting and managing expenses.

Navigating senior living with diabetes involves addressing the specific challenges associated with assisted living facilities, nursing homes, travel, and financial considerations. By actively collaborating with healthcare professionals, facility staff, and support networks, seniors can tailor their diabetes management plans to align with their changing living situations. Additionally, proactive planning, communication, and exploring available resources contribute to a comprehensive and empowered approach to diabetes care in various senior living scenarios. As seniors navigate the intersection of diabetes management and living arrangements, a holistic and well-informed strategy ensures continuity in care and promotes their overall well-being.

Chapter 9:

Aging Gracefully with Diabetes: Lifestyle and Self-Care

As seniors navigate the journey of aging with diabetes, embracing a holistic approach to lifestyle and self-care becomes paramount. This chapter explores strategies for promoting healthy aging, the crucial connection between sleep and diabetes, and the delicate balance between independence, relationships, and effective diabetes management.

9.1 Promoting Healthy Aging and Quality of Life

Aging gracefully with diabetes involves cultivating a lifestyle that prioritizes overall health and well-being. This section delves into strategies for healthy aging, emphasizing the integration of physical, mental, and emotional aspects of life.

Physical Well-being:

1. **Regular Exercise:** Engaging in regular physical activity is fundamental to healthy aging. Seniors with diabetes should incorporate exercises such as walking, swimming, or gentle yoga into their routine, tailored to their fitness levels.

2. **Balanced Nutrition:** Maintaining a balanced and nutritious diet is crucial for seniors with diabetes. Emphasizing whole foods, fiber-rich options, and adequate hydration contributes to stable blood sugar levels and overall health.

3. **Regular Health Check-ups:** Scheduling regular health check-ups ensures proactive management of diabetes-related issues. Seniors should monitor blood sugar levels, blood pressure, cholesterol, and other relevant health markers.

4. **Medication Adherence:** Consistent adherence to prescribed medications is essential. Seniors should work closely with healthcare professionals to understand the importance of medications and follow recommended dosages.

Mental and Emotional Well-being:

1. **Mindfulness Practices:** Incorporating mindfulness practices, such as meditation and deep breathing exercises, promotes mental well-being. Seniors can cultivate mindfulness to manage stress and enhance overall emotional resilience.

2. **Social Engagement:** Maintaining social connections is vital for mental health. Seniors should actively participate in social activities, fostering relationships with friends, family, and community members.

3. **Cognitive Stimulation:** Engaging in activities that stimulate the mind, such as puzzles, reading, or learning new skills, supports cognitive health. Seniors should prioritize activities that challenge and stimulate their mental faculties.

4. **Embracing Creativity:** Exploring creative outlets, such as art, music, or writing, provides a positive channel for self-expression. Seniors can embrace creative pursuits to enhance their emotional well-being.

Preventive Health Measures:

1. **Immunizations:** Staying up-to-date with vaccinations is crucial for preventing illnesses. Seniors with diabetes should receive recommended immunizations, including flu shots and pneumonia vaccines.

2. **Bone Health:** Ensuring adequate calcium and vitamin D intake supports bone health. Seniors should discuss bone health with their healthcare professionals, exploring supplements if needed.

3. **Vision and Hearing Checks:** Regular vision and hearing checks contribute to overall health. Seniors should address any changes in vision or hearing promptly to maintain a high quality of life.

4. **Fall Prevention:** Implementing measures to prevent falls, such as home modifications and balance exercises, is essential. Seniors should be proactive in maintaining a safe environment to minimize the risk of falls.

9.2 Sleep and Diabetes: Importance and Strategies for Restful Sleep

Quality sleep plays a significant role in overall health and diabetes management. This section explores the importance of sleep for seniors with diabetes and provides strategies for ensuring restful and rejuvenating sleep.

Understanding the Connection:

1. **Impact of Diabetes on Sleep:** Diabetes can influence sleep patterns. Seniors may experience challenges

such as insomnia, sleep apnea, or restless leg syndrome, impacting the overall quality of sleep.

2. **Reciprocal Relationship:** The relationship between diabetes and sleep is reciprocal. Poor sleep can affect blood sugar control, and uncontrolled diabetes may contribute to sleep disturbances. Seniors should recognize the interplay between the two and prioritize sleep hygiene.

3. **Hormonal Influence:** Hormonal changes associated with aging and diabetes can influence sleep. Seniors should be aware of these factors and take steps to address them for improved sleep quality.

Strategies for Restful Sleep:

1. **Consistent Sleep Schedule:** Establishing a consistent sleep schedule is crucial. Seniors should aim for a regular bedtime and wake-up time to regulate their internal body clock.

2. **Creating a Relaxing Bedtime Routine:** Engaging in relaxing activities before bedtime signals the body to prepare for sleep. Seniors can incorporate activities such as reading, gentle stretching, or listening to calming music.

3. **Optimizing Sleep Environment:** Creating a conducive sleep environment enhances restfulness. Seniors should ensure a comfortable mattress, minimal light and noise, and a cool room temperature for optimal sleep conditions.

4. **Limiting Stimulants:** Caffeine and nicotine can interfere with sleep. Seniors should limit the

consumption of stimulants, especially in the hours leading up to bedtime.

5. **Managing Stress and Anxiety:** Stress and anxiety can disrupt sleep patterns. Seniors should incorporate stress management techniques, such as mindfulness or deep breathing exercises, into their daily routine.

6. **Addressing Sleep Disorders:** Seniors experiencing persistent sleep disturbances should consult with healthcare professionals. Conditions such as sleep apnea or insomnia may require specific interventions for improved sleep quality.

9.3 Balancing Independence, Relationships, and Diabetes Management

Maintaining independence and nurturing relationships are integral aspects of a fulfilling senior life. This section explores the delicate balance between autonomy, social connections, and effective diabetes management.

Promoting Independence:

1. **Personalized Diabetes Management Plans:** Seniors should work with healthcare professionals to create personalized diabetes management plans that align with their lifestyle and goals. This facilitates independence in daily diabetes care.

2. **Assistive Devices and Technologies:** Leveraging assistive devices and technologies enhances independence. Seniors can explore tools such as glucose monitors, insulin pens, and medication reminders to streamline diabetes management.

3. **Self-Monitoring Practices:** Regular self-monitoring of blood sugar levels empowers seniors in their diabetes management. Understanding the impact of lifestyle choices on blood sugar levels promotes informed decision-making.

4. **Mobility and Accessibility:** Maintaining mobility and accessibility is essential for independence. Seniors should address any mobility concerns promptly and make modifications to living spaces to ensure ease of movement.

Nurturing Relationships:

1. **Effective Communication:** Open communication with loved ones about diabetes management fosters understanding and support. Seniors should share their needs, challenges, and successes, creating a supportive environment.

2. **Family Involvement:** Involving family members in diabetes care promotes a collaborative approach. Seniors can designate specific roles, share information about their diabetes management plan, and engage family members in supportive activities.

3. **Social Engagement:** Balancing diabetes management with social activities is crucial. Seniors should actively participate in social events, gatherings, and community activities while ensuring that their diabetes care remains a priority.

4. **Supportive Friendships:** Cultivating supportive friendships contributes to emotional well-being. Seniors can build relationships with individuals who

understand and respect their diabetes management needs.

Navigating Social Situations:

1. **Managing Food Choices:** Seniors can navigate social situations by making mindful food choices. Communicating dietary preferences and restrictions ensures that they can enjoy social events while prioritizing their health.

2. **Educating Others:** Educating friends and acquaintances about diabetes fosters a supportive environment. Seniors can share information about diabetes, its management, and any specific considerations relevant to social interactions.

3. **Advocating for Needs:** Advocating for one's needs is essential in social situations. Seniors should feel empowered to communicate their requirements, such as the availability of water, breaks for blood sugar checks, or considerations for meal timing.

Aging gracefully with diabetes involves embracing a lifestyle that prioritizes physical, mental, and emotional well-being. By promoting healthy aging strategies, recognizing the importance of sleep, and balancing independence with relationships, seniors can navigate the complexities of aging with resilience and positivity. This chapter encourages seniors to actively engage in self-care practices, communicate effectively with their support networks, and approach aging with diabetes as a journey of continuous growth and fulfillment. Through proactive management and a holistic approach, seniors can age with grace, maintaining a high quality of life while effectively managing their diabetes.

Conclusion:

Embracing Life's Journey with Diabetes as a Senior

Navigating life's journey with diabetes as a senior is a profound and transformative experience that requires resilience, adaptability, and a commitment to holistic well-being. This concluding reflection encapsulates the essence of embracing the challenges and joys of living with diabetes in the senior years, emphasizing the importance of a positive mindset, proactive management, and a supportive community.

The Resilience of the Human Spirit:

1. **Facing Challenges with Resilience:** Seniors living with diabetes embody the resilience of the human spirit. The challenges posed by diabetes, from daily management to potential health complications, are met with a steadfast determination to overcome obstacles and thrive.

2. **Adapting to Change:** Embracing life's journey involves adapting to the inevitable changes that come with aging and managing a chronic condition. Seniors with diabetes showcase remarkable adaptability, adjusting lifestyles, routines, and priorities to ensure a fulfilling and balanced existence.

The Positive Mindset:

1. **Focusing on Positivity:** A positive mindset is a powerful tool in the journey with diabetes. Seniors who approach each day with optimism, viewing challenges

as opportunities for growth, cultivate a mental environment that supports overall well-being.

2. **Celebrating Achievements:** Recognizing and celebrating achievements, whether big or small, is integral to maintaining a positive outlook. Seniors can take pride in their commitment to diabetes management, acknowledging the progress made on their unique paths.

Proactive Management and Empowerment:

1. **Active Engagement in Self-Care:** Seniors actively engage in self-care, recognizing the significance of their role in managing diabetes. From monitoring blood sugar levels to making lifestyle choices that promote health, the empowerment derived from proactive management is transformative.

2. **Collaboration with Healthcare Professionals:** The partnership between seniors and healthcare professionals underscores the importance of collaborative care. Through open communication, shared decision-making, and a commitment to mutual goals, seniors and their healthcare teams work together to optimize health outcomes.

Building a Supportive Community:

1. **The Role of Support Networks:** Life's journey with diabetes is enriched by supportive networks. Whether it's family, friends, or fellow seniors facing similar challenges, the collective strength of a supportive community provides comfort, understanding, and encouragement.

2. **Advocating for Support:** Seniors actively advocate for the support they need. By fostering open communication with loved ones and healthcare professionals, they create an environment where their needs are understood and met, contributing to a sense of empowerment.

Reflections on Growth and Wisdom:

1. **Continuous Growth:** Embracing life's journey with diabetes as a senior is synonymous with continuous growth. Each day presents opportunities to learn, adapt, and refine strategies for optimal diabetes management, contributing to personal and emotional growth.

2. **Wisdom Through Experience:** Seniors bring a wealth of wisdom to their diabetes journey. Through years of experience, they develop insights into their bodies, effective management techniques, and a profound understanding of the interconnectedness between physical and emotional well-being.

The Beauty of a Balanced Life:

1. **Prioritizing a Balanced Lifestyle:** Seniors with diabetes find beauty in the balance between health and life's other aspects. They appreciate the importance of maintaining a balance between diabetes management and the pursuit of passions, relationships, and meaningful experiences.

2. **Celebrating Life's Joys:** Amidst the challenges, seniors find joy in the everyday moments. Whether it's sharing a meal with loved ones, engaging in hobbies, or

savoring the beauty of nature, they celebrate the richness of life while managing diabetes with grace.

Embracing life's journey with diabetes as a senior is a testament to the strength of the human spirit and the capacity for growth and resilience. It is a journey marked by positive perspectives, proactive management, and the invaluable support of communities and healthcare professionals. Seniors navigate this path with wisdom, continuously adapting to the ebb and flow of life while savoring its joys. Through their unique experiences and journeys, seniors with diabetes contribute not only to their well-being but also to a broader narrative of inspiration and empowerment for others facing similar challenges.

Glossary

1. **Blood Glucose Levels:** The concentration of glucose (sugar) present in the bloodstream. It is a key parameter monitored by individuals with diabetes to manage their condition effectively.

2. **Diabetes Mellitus:** A chronic medical condition characterized by elevated blood sugar levels resulting from the body's inability to produce or effectively use insulin. There are different types of diabetes, including Type 1, Type 2, and gestational diabetes.

3. **Insulin:** A hormone produced by the pancreas that regulates blood sugar by facilitating the uptake of glucose into cells. People with diabetes may require insulin injections to manage their blood glucose levels.

4. **Type 1 Diabetes:** A form of diabetes characterized by the immune system attacking and destroying the insulin-producing beta cells in the pancreas. Individuals with Type 1 diabetes need insulin therapy for survival.

5. **Type 2 Diabetes:** A condition where the body becomes resistant to insulin or fails to produce enough insulin to maintain normal blood sugar levels. Lifestyle changes, medications, and sometimes insulin are used to manage Type 2 diabetes.

6. **Gestational Diabetes:** Diabetes that occurs during pregnancy and can lead to complications for both the mother and baby. It usually resolves after childbirth, but it increases the risk of developing Type 2 diabetes later in life.

7. **Hypoglycemia:** A condition characterized by abnormally low blood sugar levels, often resulting from excessive insulin or certain medications. Symptoms may include shakiness, dizziness, sweating, and confusion.

8. **Hyperglycemia:** Elevated blood sugar levels, are a common concern for individuals with diabetes. It can lead to symptoms such as increased thirst, frequent urination, and fatigue if not properly managed.

9. **A1C Test:** A blood test that provides an average blood sugar level over the past two to three months. It is a key indicator of long-term glucose control in individuals with diabetes.

10. **Carbohydrates:** One of the three macronutrients, along with protein and fat, found in food. Carbohydrates are broken down into glucose, impacting blood sugar levels and requiring careful monitoring for individuals with diabetes.

11. **Hemoglobin:** A protein in red blood cells that binds to oxygen. The A1C test measures the percentage of hemoglobin that is glycated, providing insight into average blood sugar levels over time.

12. **Ketones:** Chemical substances produced when the body breaks down fat for energy in the absence of sufficient insulin. Elevated ketone levels can lead to a serious condition called diabetic ketoacidosis (DKA).

13. **Complications:** Long-term health issues that can arise from uncontrolled diabetes, including cardiovascular

disease, kidney damage, nerve damage, and vision problems.

14. **Continuous Glucose Monitoring (CGM):** A system that continuously tracks blood sugar levels throughout the day and night, providing real-time data to help individuals with diabetes manage their condition more effectively.

15. **Insulin Resistance:** A condition where cells in the body do not respond effectively to insulin, leading to elevated blood sugar levels. It is a common feature of Type 2 diabetes.

16. **Pancreas:** An organ located behind the stomach that plays a crucial role in digestion and blood sugar regulation. It produces insulin and other enzymes necessary for the breakdown of food.

17. **Polypharmacy:** The use of multiple medications to manage various health conditions. Seniors with diabetes may be prescribed multiple medications to address the complexities of their health needs.

18. **Retinopathy:** A diabetes-related complication that affects the eyes, potentially leading to vision loss. Regular eye exams are crucial for detecting and managing retinopathy.

19. **Neuropathy:** Nerve damage often associated with diabetes, leading to symptoms such as numbness, tingling, and pain, particularly in the extremities.

20. **Endocrinologist:** A medical doctor specializing in the diagnosis and treatment of hormonal disorders, including diabetes.

THE END

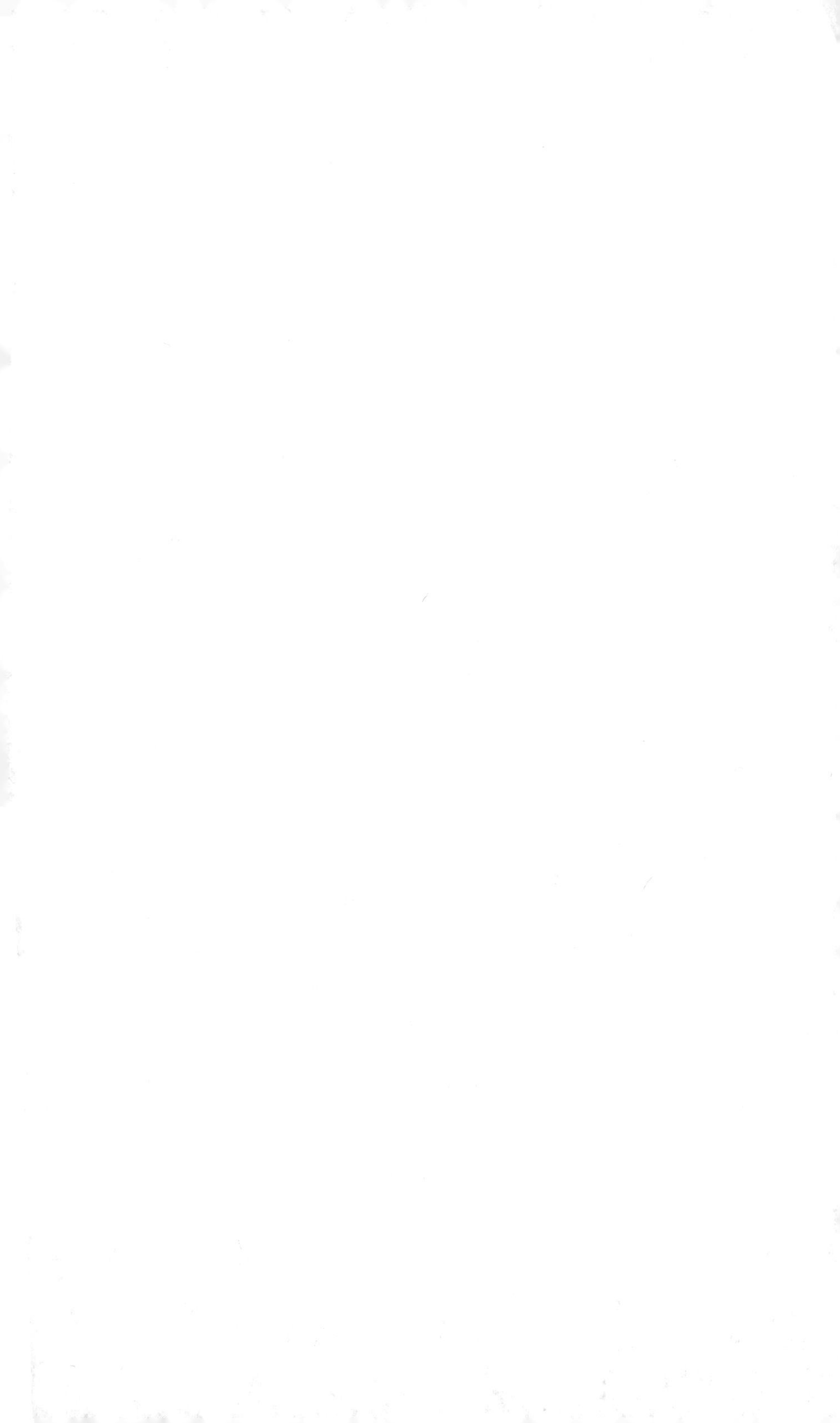